SPORTS INJURIES

Edited & Compiled by

Dr. R.V.S. Reddy P.S.A.
M.A. (Physical Education), M.Phil., Ph.D.,
Lecturer & H.O.D. (Physical Education)
N.W.W. Society's College of Physical Education
Karnataka

SPORTS PUBLICATION
7/26, Ground Floor, Ansari Road,
Darya Ganj, New Delhi-110002
Phones: (Office) 65749511 (Fax) 011-23240261
(Mobile) 9868028838 (Residence) 27562163
E-mail: lakshaythani@hotmail.com

Published by:

SPORTS PUBLICATION
7/26, Ground Floor, Ansari Road, Darya Ganj, New Delhi-110002
Ph. : (Office) 65749511, 23240261 (Mobile) 9868028838
(Residence) 27562163 (Fax) 011-23240261
E-mail: *lakshaythani@hotmail.com*

I.S.B.N: 978-81-7879-548-5

PRINTED IN INDIA 2009

Laser Typeset by:
JAIN MEDIA GRAPHICS,
C-4/95-A, Keshav Puram, Delhi-35 Ph.: 9911151534, 9350556511, 20296366

Printed by:
CHAWLA OFFSET PRINTERS, Delhi-110052

Price: Rs. 400/-

CONTENTS

1

Basic Concept of Sports Injuries

Sports injuries are injuries that occur to athletes in major sporting events. In many cases, these types of injuries are due to overuse of a part of the body when participating in a certain activity. For example, runner's knee is a painful condition generally associated with running, while tennis elbow is a form of repetitive stress injury at the elbow, although it does not often occur with tennis players. Other types of injuries can be caused by a hard contact with something. This can often cause a broken bone or torn ligament or tendon.

Injuries are a common occurrence in professional sports and most teams have a staff of Athletic Trainers and close connections to the medical community. Controversy has arisen at times when teams have made decisions that could threaten a players long-term health for short term gain.

It is inevitable that injuries will always be associated with physical activity and athletics. The risk of injury is much higher in some sports, such as those requiring contact or collision, but is inherent to all athletic activity. Although the majority of athletic injuries are relatively minor, the potential for serious and passible life-threatening injuries is constantly present. The incidence of serious and life-threatening conditions associated with athletic activity has decreased over the last several years as a result of the delineation of causative factors and subsequent rule modifications in many sports and vast improvements and increased sophistication in all facets of sports medicine and athletic training.

In spite of this increased sophistication, there has been an overall increase in the number of athletic injuries; this is primarily the result of an increase in the number of participants, the intensity of modern training techniques and the expansion of athletic activities. Today a wider selection of athletic activities, physical fitness programs and sports are available to a larger cross-section of the population than ever before.

Interest in physical activities and athletics continues to increase and participation in no longer limited to high school, college, amateur, and professional athletes. A greater number of organized athletic programs are available to children in junior high school and upper elementary grades. Youth sports competition, recreational programs, intramural activities, and sports for the handicapped and all age groups are increasing in popularity.

The number of participants in all areas continues to increase dramatically. The development of many women's athletic programs is another factor that has greatly changed the number of sports activities and opportunities for participation. Because of all these developments, there are greater opportunities for persons of all ages to participate in recreational and competitive activities. People are becoming more health and fitness conscious than ever before.

The awareness has produced an increased interest

in the benefits of physical fitness. More people than ever before are participating in life-time activities such as walking, jogging, bicycling, swimming, golf, and tennis. People today have more leisure time available as a result of many factors, including shorter work weeks, mechanization, and time-saving devices. Many people are using this additional leisure time to participate in recreational activities requiring some degree of physical exertion.

Whatever the reason for the dramatic increase in the number of participants and activities available, injuries are a reality at every level of participation and in every type of program. Participants in all forms of athletic activity are subjected to many stresses and forces that can result in injury. It is important to remember that injuries to athletes are essentially no different from those suffered by nonathletes.

A sprained ankle can result in the same severity of damage whether it is sustained by a competitive athlete ora week-end jogger. However, the demands in terms of evaluation, treatment, rehabilitation, and return to activity are usually significantly greater for the competitive athlete.

SPORTS MEDICINE

Just as there have been tremendous increases in participation and interest in athletics, there have been corresponding increases in interest, knowledge, and understanding concerning all aspects of the medical management of athletes and athletic injuries.

A new phrase has been coined to describe this vast network of medical management: sports medicine. Sports medicine encompasses all phases of medical concerns relating to the athlete: biomechanical, psychological, nutritional, environmental, pathological, and physiological. The field of sports medicine has seen phenomenal development in recent years, as evidenced by the professional associations designating sports medicine as a speciality, the vast amounts of literature, research, and educational experiences now available, and the number of medical clinics specializing in sports medicine emerging throughout the country.

Sports medicine is a rapidly growing, dynamic field. The knowledge and techniques gained are benefiting not only competitive athletes and the vast legion of fitness buffs but also everyone else involved in athletic and non-athletic activities. Sports medicine includes all medical and para-medical professionals who are concerned with and provide expertise aimed at improving the performance and the health care of athletes. One of the subspecializations of sports medicine is athletic training.

ATHLETIC TRAINING

As a sports medicine subspeciality, athletic training provides a wide array of health care support services for athletes. Athletic training as defined by the National Athletic Trainer's Association is "the art and science of prevention and management of injuries at all levels of athletic activity". The provider of athletic training services is an athletic trainer.

The profession of athletic training and the position of the athletic trainer on the sports medicine team have developed to meet a demand for someone highly skilled in the evaluation, management, and care of athletic injuries. As long as there has been athletics, there has generally been someone designated to manage or care for athletes who become injured.

In the past this position of responsibility was generally filled by a coach, teacher, student, or other interested person. Now many of these positions at the collegiate and professional levels are being filled by a qualified athletic trainer. However, much of the responsibility for the medical care of athletes, particularly at the high-school level, remains with the coach and will continue as such until the need for highly skilled athletic trainers is recognized.

There appears to be a need for an increase in the number and availability of qualified athletic trainers nationally. As compared with other allied health professions, athletic training is quite young. NATA was founded in 1950. The qualifications and requirements to become an athletic trainer have become more stringent over the years. In 1969 a procedure was developed for these institutions offering athletic training curricula to obtain NATA approval.

At that time only two schools were selected that met all requirements for approval. Today there are over 70 schools offering NATA-approved curricula. In 1970 a certifying procedure for athletic trainers was established and has been continually upgraded and improved. To become an athletic trainer a person must possess a college degree that fulfils specific educational and practical requirements. On successful completion of these requirements the candidate must then take a national certifying examination designed to ensure that he or she meets the minimal standards and competencies required to become an athletic trainer.

In addition to obtaining the initial certification, athletic trainers must also earn a designated number of continuing education units to maintain their certified status. Today's athletic trainer is more than just a technician designated to tape ankles, apply bandages, or "rubdown" athletes. Athletic training is becoming more scientific, and athletic trainers are more knowledgeable about the many aspects of health care for athletes. The athletic trainer has become a vital member of the sports medicine team.

In addition to the athletic trainer, this team includes the team physician, coach, and other professionals involved in providing health care for athletes. It is the athletic trainer's responsibility to coordinate the health care services available. In 1982 a role delineation study conducted by the NATA classified the duties or functions of an athletic trainer into six major categories:

(1) prevention

(2) assessment,

(3) treatment, management, and disposition,

(4) rehabilitation,

(5) organization and administration, and

(6) education and counselling of injured athletes.

Each of these areas is important and all are interrelated. The athletic trainer must develop knowledge and competency in each category to provide athletes with optimal medical care. The athletic trainer muse be able to combine medical and scientific information in the areas of anatomy, physiology, kinesiology, psychology, physiology of exercise, health, physics, nutrition, and first aid with a wide array of complex practical skills.

In addition, he or she must also have a sincere

interest in athletics and in working with athletes and must possess communication and leadership skills. The athletic trainer is no longer a "jack of all trades, master of none". He or she is a professional who must be proficient in many varied skills.

ASSESSMENT

Athletic trainers must possess a high level of proficiency in assessment skills to accurately recognize and evaluate the nature and severity of an athletic injury. Athletic trainers are normally at the location or playing field where an injury occurs and will have to handle the emergency care. They must be able to recognize and deal with such conditions as severe head or spine injuries, haemorrhaging, shock, heat illness, or choking.

Athletic trainers must be prepared to administer cardiopulmonary resuscitation, apply emergency splinting, or supervise the transportation of an injured athlete. The athletic injury assessment process is based on a scientific method that involves:

(a) recognition and statement of the problem,

(b) creation and testing of hypotheses to solve the solve the problem,

(c) collection of data about the problem.

An athletic trainer's initial assessment creates the foundation or data base for the ensuing procedures. It begins with the collection of data related to the injury through the systematic steps of history, observation, palpation, and stress manoeuvres. From the data collected, the athletic trainer must determine and initiate the appropriate course of action. This includes emergency medical care, follow-up treatment procedures, transportation, medical referral, rehabilitation strategies, or return to athletic activity.

Once action has been taken, the athletic trainer must continually evaluate the results of this action. Is the athletic getting better or worse? Why? What can be done to improve or enhance the athlete's recovery? The athletic trainer should then modify or adjust the plan of action accordingly. Assessment and reassessment are going processes in athletic training.

REHABILITATION

Rehabilitation is the restoration of normal form and function after an injury. Athletic rehabilitation is the reconditioning of an injured athlete to his or her highest level of function in the shortest possible time. This level of function is generally higher than that of a nonathlete. Athletic trainers must be skilled in developing programs to effectively rehabilitate an athlete in a minimal amount of time.

Depending upon the nature and the conditions surrounding the injury, rehabilitation requires a progressive, systematic program that develops range of motion, muscular strength and endurance, coordinated movements, functional activities, and circulorespirator endurance. Although each of these phases overlap, maximal development of any phases requires prior development of the preceding phase. During rehabilitation there should be repeated assessment techniques performed to evaluate progress and indicate appropriate follow-up care.

PREVENTION

The best method of managing and caring for athletic injuries is to prevent them from occurring; thus much of the athletic trainer's time and effort is devoted to preventing injuries. Numerous factors briefly discussed in this section are important in the prevention of athletic injuries. A thorough pre-participation evaluation does not guarantee that an athlete will participate injury free but it does firm that there is no discernible clinical reason to preclude participation. Proper conditioning is the preventing medicine of athletics.

Athletic trainers often work in conjunction with coaches in establishing pre-season, in-season, and post-season conditioning programs. Another facet of athletic injury prevention in which the athletic trainer is involved is the selection, fitting, and maintenance of protective equipment. An athletic trainer may also be responsible for checking the safety of facilities and apparatus required for athletic activity. More familiar preventive tasks performed by athletic trainers include the application of protective taping, padding, bandaging, braces, and other devices.

Athletic trainers must also constantly observe their athletes. If recognized early, minor problems can often be treated with minimal inconvenience to the athlete and no significant decrease in performance. Early recognition and effective treatment prevent most minor injuries from becoming more severe and disabling. An injury that is properly recognized and managed effectively generally does not become more severe, and the potential for reinjury is less.

In addition, athletic trainers are often asked to counsel athletes and coaches in the areas of diet, rest, and sanitation.

MANAGEMENT AND TREATMENT

Athletic trainers must be skilled in various

management and treatment procedures. These include:

(1) administering immediate first aid,

(2) providing therapy to promote healing, and recovery,

(3) applying protective techniques to support and protect an injured area, and

(4) referring an injured athlete for other medical assistance when necessary.

Athletic trainers can have a dramatic effect on the overall recovery of an injured athlete by the proper use of treatment procedures. The goal is to return the injured athlete to activity as soon as possible without risking further injury. The treatment of an athletic injury is a three-step process:

(1) examination of the signs and symptoms,

(2) application of treatment routines, and

(3) assessment of the effects of these techniques on the signs and symptoms of the injury.

This cycle continues throughout the treatment process; that is, assessment, treatment, and reassessment. If an athlete is no return optimum physical activity in a minimal amount of time, there can be no delay in an accurate assessment and a properly instituted treatment program.

ORGANISATION AND ADMINISTRATION

Often overlooked aspects of an athletic trainer's responsibilities are the organization and administration of the athletic training program, Athletic trainers must plan, organize, evaluate, and implement procedures and policies necessary to provide their athletes with the most effective health care available.

To aid in efficient health care delivery, athletic trainers must maintain accurate and detailed records to document injuries and treatments and other services rendered to the athletes under their care. Selecting, purchasing, maintaining, and instructing others in the use of equipment and supplies necessary for operation of a training room are also the athletic trainer's responsibilities.

EDUCATION AND COUNSELLING

The last function of an athletic trainer to be discussed is the role of education and counsellor to the athlete and student athletic trainer. Athletic trainers need to have the skill and knowledge necessary to instruct students in the competencies required to become professional athletic trainers.

This responsibility requires that the athletic trainer keep abreast of current sports medicine issues and also be able to convey this information to others. Another facet of education and counselling skills required is the athletic trainer's ability to recognize situations requiring consultation with other health care professionals regarding an athlete's social or personal problem. This involves skill in assessing an athlete's need for professional consultation and referral of the athlete to the appropriate professional.

To be effective communication skills. These communication skills enable the athletic trainer to interact with athletes, parents, coaches, administrators, physicians and other professionals concerning various health-related topics. To summarize, athletic trainer must develop knowledge and competency in each of these duties or functions to provide optimal medical care to athletes. Note that assessment or evaluation skills are listed and discussed under each of these categories. Athletic injury assessment is a necessary and extremely important skill for anyone who has medical responsibilities for athletes.

CLASSIFICATION

Sports injuries can be broadly classified as either traumatic or overuse injuries. Traumatic injuries account for most injuries in contact sports such as Football, Rugby, Australian rules football, Gaelic football and American football because of the dynamic and high collision nature of these sports. These injuries range from bruises and muscle strains, to fractures and head injuries.

A bruise or contusion is damage to small blood vessels which causes bleeding within the tissues. A muscle strain is a small tear of muscle fibers and a ligament sprain is a small tear of ligament tissue. The body's response to these sports injuries is the same in the initial five day period immediately following the traumatic incident - inflammation.

SIGNS AND SYMPTOMS

Inflammation is characterized by pain, localized swelling, heat, redness and a loss of function.

MECHANISM

All of these traumatic injuries cause damage to the cells that make up the soft tissues. The dead and damaged cells release chemicals, which initiate an inflammatory response. Small blood vessels are damaged and opened up, producing bleeding within the tissue. In the body's normal reaction, a small blood clot is formed in order to stop this bleeding and from this clot special cells (called fibroblasts) begin the healing process by laying down scar tissue.

The inflammatory stage is therefore the first phase of healing. However, too much of an inflammatory response in the early stage can mean that the healing process takes longer and a return to activity is delayed. The sports injury treatments are intended to minimize the inflammatory phase of an injury, so that the overall healing process is accelerated. intrinsic and extrinsic factors

PREVENTION

A comprehensive warm-up programme has been found to decrease injuries in soccer. Many athletes will partake in HGH Treatment for Athletic Enhancement as a way to prevent injuries.

Treatment

Sports injuries can be treated and managed by using the P.R.I.C.E.R... DR. ABC and T.O.T.A.P.S regimes:

P - Protect

R - Rest

I - Ice

C - Compression

E - Elevation

R - Referral

D - Danger

R - Response

A - Airway

B - Breathing

C - Circulation

T - Talk

O - Observe

T - Touch

A - Active movement

P - Passive movement

S - Skills test

The inflammatory stage typically lasts around 5 days and all treatment during this time is designed to address the cardinal signs of inflammation – pain, swelling, redness, heat and a loss of function.

Kinesiology tape, also known as elastic therapeutic tape, is used in therapy to treat injuries and relax overused muscles, and in rehabilitation to facilitate underused muscles. The wave pattern found on the tape's adhesive has a lifting effect on the skin which can reduce swelling and inflammation by improving circulation and reduce pain by taking pressure off pain receptors. Today Kinesiology tape is accepted by medical practitioners and athletes in Japan, the United States, Europe, South America, Australia, and other Asian countries. Kinesiology tape is just starting to be available to average consumers for the first time in 2009.

Compression sportswear is becoming very popular with both professional and amateur athletes. These garments are thought to both reduce the risk of muscle injury and speed up muscle recovery.

Portable Mild Hyperbaric Chamber 40" diameterAlthough not proven some professional athletes use hyperbaric chambers to speed healing. Hines Ward of the Steelers sent his personal hyperbaric chamber,(similar to the one pictured), to his hotel to sleep in believing it would help heal his sprained medial collateral ligament he suffered in their playoff win against the Ravens. Hines went on to play in Super Bowl XLIII.

Knee Injuries and Recovery

The knee is a core tool for an athlete; it allows football and basketball players to run, cut, and jump. Baseball players use their knees to push off when they throw. The flexibility and rotational ability of a knee is what helps make some tennis players superstars. It's difficult to return to competitive athletics after any serious injury, but knee injuries takes a lot longer to get over and often end a career. While having a good physical rehab process is very important, the athlete's ability to overcome the mental hurdles that are created with a knee injury will determine whether or not he will be the same player that he was before the injury.

The words "it's an ACL" strike fear in the heart of an athlete. The immediate mental translation is will I ever play again and if I do play will I ever be as good? Why do knee injuries cause so much fear in competitive athletes? According to the Brown University Biology and Medicine Web site, athletes in contact sports are 10 times more likely to have a serious knee injury than in non-contact sports, with knee injuries accounting for approximately a quarter of the injuries and generally taking two to three times longer to recovery than injuries to other parts of the body Knee injuries are also increasing, "over the last 15 years, ankle sprains have decreased by 86% and tibia fractures by 88%, but knee ligament injuries have increased by 172%".

What cause knee injuries and what is the prognosis for total rehabilitation? Leg bones are connected to the kneecap by four strong ligaments: Anterior Cruciate Ligament (ACL), Lateral Collateral Ligament (LCL), Medial Collateral Ligament (MCL), and Posterior Cruciate Ligament (PCL). The ACL provides stability and controls stress across the kneecap and keeps the knee from rotating too much or moving too far forward. Around 60% of ligament tears are ACL, most occurring in basketball, skiing, football and soccer. When an ACL tears it unravels like a rope and will not heal on its own. For competitive athletes treatment is almost always surgery. It normally takes 6 to 9 months to recovery from an ACL reconstruction surgery, at which point most athletes had returned to between 80% and 100% of their full level of previous play with about 90% returning to competition. After the first ACL injury, there is a 5 to 15% risk of repeated injury. MCL and LCL 'igament tears are less frequent then ACL injuries accounting for about 25% with LCL injury being much less frequent than MCL injuries. MCL injuries are normally caused when a significant force is applied to the side of the knee while the lower leg is held in a fixed position. The MCL is the only ligament that has enough of a blood supply to heal partial tears without surgery PCL injuries account for between 3% and 20% of all tears. Most often the cause is a blow to a bent leg. Because of the type of blow, PCL tears are often accompanied by ACL tears. While conservative treatment is still controversial in some sports for both PCL and MCL tears, it has proven to be as effective in returning an athlete back to his playing condition as has surgery.

Why or why not surgery? If an athlete wants to play competitively ACL tears require reconstructive surgery.

During surgery the old ACL is removed, a graft from the patellar tendon or the hamstring is prepared, holes are drilled in the tibia and femur and the graft is attached with screws to the bones. Now the tough part begins, surgery is followed by 6 to 9 months of rehabilitation. This rehabilitation is crucial to strengthen the areas surrounding the graft so that it does not fail. Athletes may accept that injuries are part of their lives and may know how to deal with physical rehabilitation, but few are prepared for the emotional pain, fear and anger that also result from injury. Athletes are used to being part of a team. When they are injured they are suddenly on their own. Their teammates will continue on but they now have a new job, physical and emotional rehabilitation of their bodies and much of the work will have to be accomplished on their own. In Sidelines, Psyched Up or Psyched Out? David Doermann describes a University of Utah pamphlet that is given to all student athletes to help them understand what to expect if they are injured. It describes the emotional process that happens when someone is injured as similar to the five stages of grief The first stage is denial. Athletes by their very nature believe that they are superior physically and therefore do not accept the fact they can be injured. When an athlete realizes an injury is real his reaction may be to isolate and blame himself. Denial is followed by anger, particularly at himself for allowing the injury to occur. During the third stage the athlete tries to make bargains with coaches, trainers or God, such as if I spend 2 hours walking every day I can play again in 2 months.

Very often these bargains are unreasonable dreams. The competitive athlete will now move to a period of depression, feeling sorry for themselves, withdrawing or simply giving up. This stage particularly can put an athlete's rehab off track. To be successful an athlete must finally get to the acceptance stage when he realizes that the only way to handle the injury is to focus on his physical rehab which could result in returning to competition. The factors that contribute the most to helping an athlete reach psychological acceptance and recovery are education, social support, psychological skill training and goal setting; traits that many athletes use in their pre-injury training.

Understanding an injury and their reaction to it helps athletes cope with the problems that naturally arrive along with the injury. Support and understanding of team mates, family and friends can also be a critical factor in recovery. Knowing and understanding how others have coped gives athletes mechanisms for starting to construct their own recoveries. While having social support that listens and appreciates the seriousness of an injury is necessary, too much sympathy from family or friends can impair the athlete's acceptance level which can slow or derail the recovery process. A study done by the Aristotle University of Thessaloniki, Greece concludes that "psychological intervention techniques can aid significantly to the rehabilitation process. In particular, the goal setting process seems to have positive clout in the athletic injury recovery, in the attitude of the injured athlete, in the successful confrontation of the injury, in the recovery of confidence and in the adherence to the rehabilitation program".

2

What Are Sports Injuries?

The term sports injury, in the broadest sense, refers to the kinds of injuries that most commonly occur during sports or exercise. Some sports injuries result from accidents; others are due to poor training practices, improper equipment, lack of conditioning, or insufficient warmup and stretching.

Although virtually any part of your body can be injured during sports or exercise, the term is usually reserved for injuries that involve the musculoskeletal system, which includes the muscles, bones, and associated tissues like cartilage. Traumatic brain and spinal cord injuries, (relatively rare during sports or exercise) and bruises are considered briefly in the appendix. Following are some of the most common sports injuries.

SPRAINS AND STRAINS

A sprain is a stretch or tear of a ligament, the band of connective tissues that joins the end of one bone with another. Sprains are caused by trauma such as a fall or blow to the body that knocks a joint out of position and, in the worst case, ruptures the supporting ligaments. Sprains can range from first degree (minimally stretched ligament) to third degree (a complete tear). Areas of the body most vulnerable to sprains are ankles, knees, and wrists. Signs of a sprain include varying degrees of tenderness or pain; bruising; inflammation; swelling; inability to move a limb or joint; or joint looseness, laxity, or instability.

A strain is a twist, pull, or tear of a muscle or tendon, a cord of tissue connecting muscle to bone. It is an acute, noncontact injury that results from overstretching or overcontraction. Symptoms of a strain include pain, muscle spasm, and loss of strength. Although it's hard to tell the difference between mild and moderate strains, severe strains not treated professionally can cause damage and loss of function.

KNEE INJURIES

Because of its complex structure and weight-bearing capacity, the knee is the most commonly injured joint. Each year, more than 5.5 million people visit doctors for knee problems.

Knee injuries can range from mild to severe. Some of the less severe, yet still painful and functionally limiting, knee problems are runner's knee (pain or tenderness close to or under the knee cap at the front or side of the knee), iliotibial band syndrome (pain on the outer side of the knee), and tendinitis, also called tendinosis (marked by degeneration within a tendon, usually where it joins the bone).

More severe injuries include bone bruises or damage to the cartilage or ligaments. There are two types of cartilage in the knee. One is the meniscus, a crescent-shaped disc that absorbs shock between the thigh (femur) and lower leg bones (tibia and fibula). The other is a surface-coating (or articular) cartilage. It covers the ends of the bones where they meet, allowing them to glide against one another. The four major ligaments that support the knee are the anterior cruciate ligament

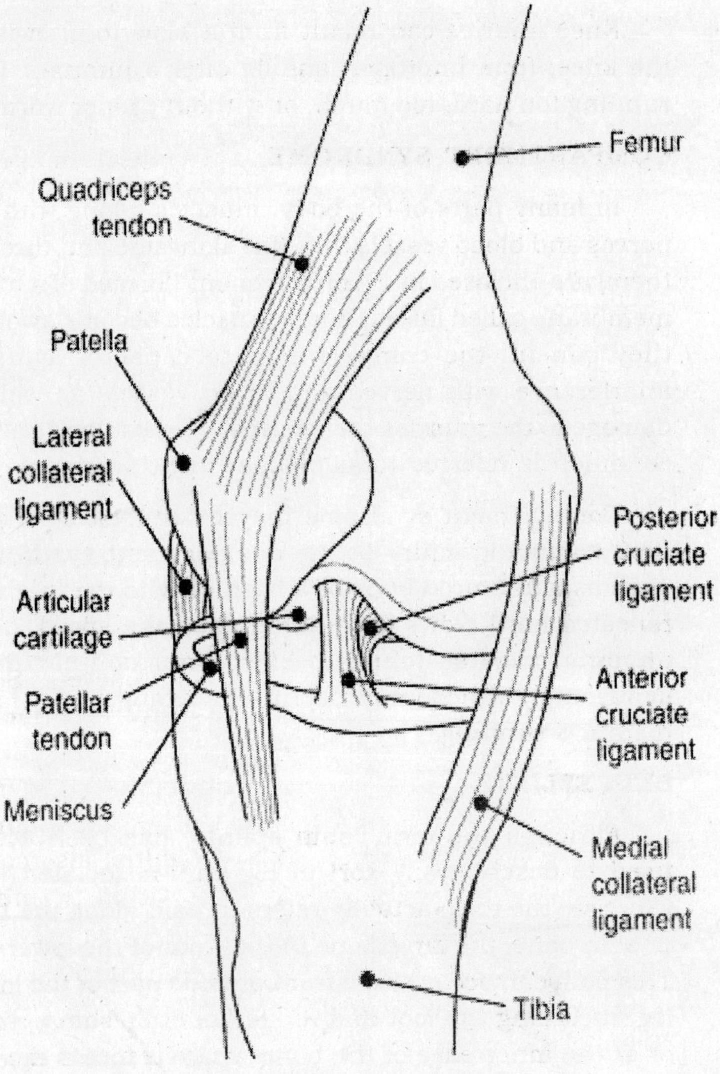

LATERAL VIEW OF THE KNEE

(ACL), the posterior cruciate ligament (PCL), the medial collateral ligament (MCL), and the lateral collateral ligament (LCL).

Knee injuries can result from a blow to or twist of the knee; from improper landing after a jump; or from running too hard, too much, or without proper warmup.

COMPARTMENT SYNDROME

In many parts of the body, muscles (along with the nerves and blood vessels that run alongside and through them) are enclosed in a "compartment" formed of a tough membrane called fascia. When muscles become swollen, they can fill the compartment to capacity, causing interference with nerves and blood vessels as well as damage to the muscles themselves. The resulting painful condition is referred to as compartment syndrome.

Compartment syndrome may be caused by a one-time traumatic injury (acute compartment syndrome), such as a fractured bone or a hard blow to the thigh, by repeated hard blows (depending upon the sport), or by ongoing overuse (chronic exertional compartment syndrome), which may occur, for example, in long-distance running.

SHIN SPLINTS

Although the term "shin splints" has been widely used to describe any sort of leg pain associated with exercise, the term actually refers to pain along the tibia or shin bone, the large bone in the front of the lower leg. This pain can occur at the front outside part of the lower leg, including the foot and ankle (anterior shin splints) or at the inner edge of the bone where it meets the calf muscles (medial shin splints).

Shin splints are primarily seen in runners, particularly those just starting a running program. Risk factors for shin splints include overuse or incorrect use of the lower leg; improper stretching, warmup, or exercise technique; overtraining; running or jumping on hard surfaces; and running in shoes that don't have enough support. These injuries are often associated with flat (overpronated) feet.

ACHILLES TENDON INJURIES

An Achilles tendon injury results from a stretch, tear, or irritation to the tendon connecting the calf muscle to the back of the heel. These injuries can be so sudden

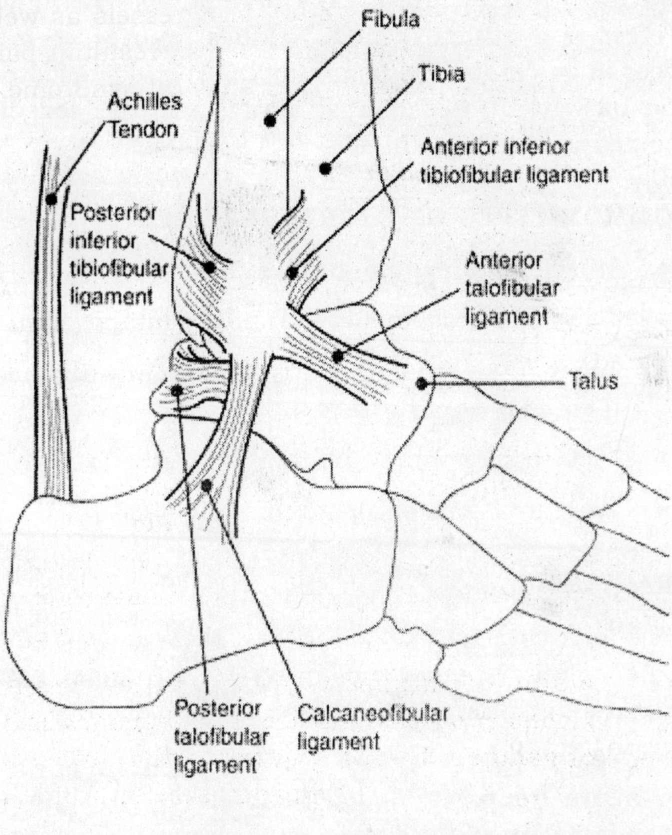

LATERAL VIEW OF THE ANKLE

and agonizing that they have been known to bring down charging professional football players in shocking fashion.

The most common cause of Achilles tendon tears is a problem called tendinitis, a degenerative condition caused by aging or overuse. When a tendon is weakened, trauma can cause it to rupture.

Achilles tendon injuries are common in middle-aged "weekend warriors" who may not exercise regularly or take time to stretch properly before an activity. Among professional athletes, most Achilles injuries seem to occur in quick-acceleration, jumping sports like football and basketball, and almost always end the season's competition for the athlete.

COMMON TYPES OF SPORTS INJURIES

- Muscle sprains and strains
- Tears of the ligaments that hold joints together
- Tears of the tendons that support joints and allow them to move
- Dislocated joints
- Fractured bones, including vertebrae.

FRACTURES

A fracture is a break in the bone that can occur from either a quick, one-time injury to the bone (acute fracture) or from repeated stress to the bone over time (stress fracture).

Acute fractures: Acute fractures can be simple (a clean break with little damage to the surrounding tissue) or compound (a break in which the bone pierces the skin with little damage to the surrounding tissue). Most acute fractures are emergencies. One that breaks the skin is especially dangerous because there is a high risk of infection.

Stress fractures: Stress fractures occur largely in the feet and legs and are common in sports that require repetitive impact, primarily running/jumping sports such as gymnastics or track and field. Running creates forces two to three times a person's body weight on the lower limbs.

The most common symptom of a stress fracture is pain at the site that worsens with weight-bearing activity. Tenderness and swelling often accompany the pain.

DISLOCATIONS

When the two bones that come together to form a joint become separated, the joint is described as being dislocated. Contact sports such as football and basketball, as well as high-impact sports and sports that can result in excessive stretching or falling, cause the majority of dislocations. A dislocated joint is an emergency situation that requires medical treatment.

THE SHOULDER JOINT

The joints most likely to be dislocated are some of the hand joints. Aside from these joints, the joint most frequently dislocated is the shoulder. Dislocations of the knees, hips, and elbows are uncommon.

WHAT'S THE DIFFERENCE BETWEEN ACUTE AND CHRONIC INJURIES?

Regardless of the specific structure affected, sports injuries can generally be classified in one of two ways: acute or chronic.

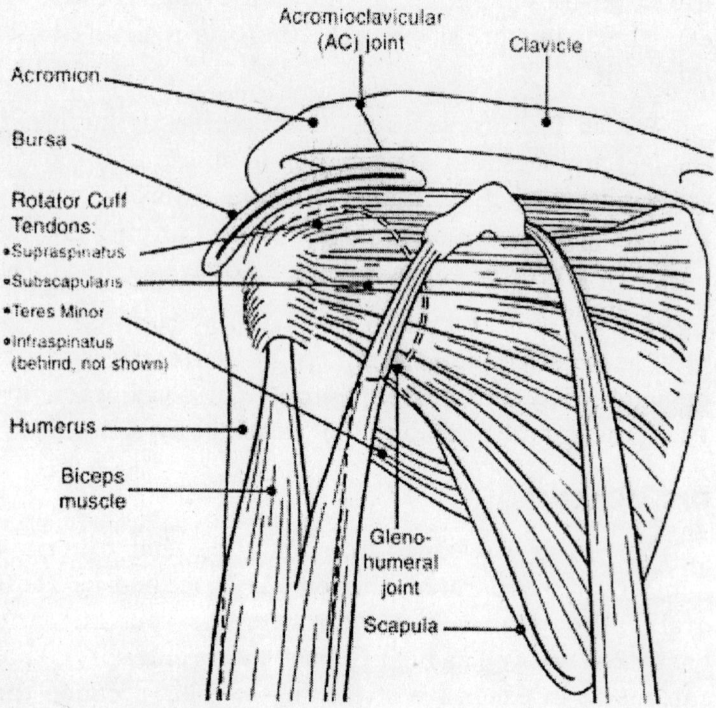

ACUTE INJURIES

Acute injuries, such as a sprained ankle, strained back, or fractured hand, occur suddenly during activity. Signs of an acute injury include the following:

- sudden, severe pain
- swelling
- inability to place weight on a lower limb
- extreme tenderness in an upper limb
- inability to move a joint through its full range of motion
- extreme limb weakness

- visible dislocation or break of a bone.

CHRONIC INJURIES

Chronic injuries usually result from overusing one area of the body while playing a sport or exercising over a long period. The following are signs of a chronic injury:

- pain when performing an activity
- a dull ache when at rest
- swelling.

WHAT SHOULD I DO IF I SUFFER AN INJURY?

Whether an injury is acute or chronic, there is never a good reason to try to "work through" the pain of an injury. When you have pain from a particular movement or activity, STOP! Continuing the activity only causes further harm.

Some injuries require prompt medical attention (see "Who Should I See for My Injury?"), while others can be self-treated. Here's what you need to know about both types:

When to Seek Medical Treatment

You should call a health professional if:

- The injury causes severe pain, swelling, or numbness.
- You can't tolerate any weight on the area.
- The pain or dull ache of an old injury is accompanied by increased swelling or joint abnormality or instability.

To learn about treating sports injuries.

WHEN AND HOW TO TREAT AT HOME

If you don't have any of the above symptoms, it's probably safe to treat the injury at home—at least at first. If pain or other symptoms worsen, it's best to check with your health care provider. Use the RICE method to relieve pain and inflammation and speed healing. Follow these four steps immediately after injury and continue for at least 48 hours.

Rest. Reduce regular exercise or activities of daily living as needed. If you cannot put weight on an ankle or knee, crutches may help. If you use a cane or one crutch for an ankle injury, use it on the uninjured side to help you lean away and relieve weight on the injured ankle.

Ice. Apply an ice pack to the injured area for 20 minutes at a time, four to eight times a day. A cold pack, ice bag, or plastic bag filled with crushed ice and wrapped in a towel can be used. To avoid cold injury and frostbite, do not apply the ice for more than 20 minutes. (Note: Do not use heat immediately after an injury. This tends to increase internal bleeding or swelling. Heat can be used later on to relieve muscle tension and promote relaxation.)

Compression. Compression of the injured area may help reduce swelling. Compression can be achieved with elastic wraps, special boots, air casts, and splints. Ask your health care provider for advice on which one to use.

Elevation. If possible, keep the injured ankle, knee, elbow, or wrist elevated on a pillow, above the level of the heart, to help decrease swelling.

The Body's Healing Process

From the moment a bone breaks or a ligament tears,

your body goes to work to repair the damage. Here s what happens at each stage of the healing process:

At the moment of injury: Chemicals are released from damaged cells, triggering a process called inflammation. Blood vessels at the injury site become dilated; blood flow increases to carry nutrients to the site of tissue damage.

Within hours of injury: White blood cells (leukocytes) travel down the bloodstream to the injury site where they begin to tear down and remove damaged tissue, allowing other specialized cells to start developing scar tissue.

Within days of injury: Scar tissue is formed on the skin or inside the body. The amount of scarring may be proportional to the amount of swelling, inflammation, or bleeding within. In the next few weeks, the damaged area will regain a great deal of strength as scar tissue continues to form.

Within a month of injury: Scar tissue may start to shrink, bringing damaged, torn, or separated tissues back together. However, it may be several months or more before the injury is completely healed.

Who Should I See for My Injury?

Although severe injuries will need to be seen immediately in an emergency room, particularly if they occur on the weekend or after office hours, most sports injuries can be evaluated and, in many cases, treated by your primary health care provider.

Depending on your preference and the severity of your injury or the likelihood that your injury may cause ongoing, long-term problems, you may want to see, or have your primary health care professional refer you to, one of the following:

Orthopaedic surgeon: A doctor specializing in the diagnosis and treatment of the musculoskeletal system, which includes bones, joints, ligaments, tendons, muscles, and nerves.

Physical therapist/physiotherapist: A health care professional who can develop a rehabilitation program. Your primary care physician may refer you to a physical therapist after you begin to recover from your injury to help strengthen muscles and joints and prevent further injury.

How Are Sports Injuries Treated?

Although using the RICE technique described previously can be helpful for any sports injury, RICE is often just a starting point. Here are some other treatments your doctor or other health care provider may administer, recommend, or prescribe to help your injury heal.

Nonsteroidal Anti-Inflammatory Drugs (NSAIDs)

The moment you are injured, chemicals are released from damaged tissue cells. This triggers the first stage of healing: inflammation (see "The Body's Healing Process" box). Inflammation causes tissues to become swollen, tender, and painful. Although inflammation is needed for healing, it can actually slow the healing process if left unchecked.

To reduce inflammation and pain, doctors and other health care providers often recommend taking an over-the-counter (OTC) nonsteroidal anti-inflammatory drug (NSAID) such as aspirin, ibuprofen (Advil,1 Motrin IB, Nuprin), ketoprofen (Actron, Orudis KT), or naproxen sodium (Aleve). For more severe pain and inflammation, doctors may prescribe one of several dozen NSAIDs available in prescription strength.2

Brand names included in this booklet are provided as examples only, and their inclusion does not mean that these products are endorsed by the National Institutes of Health or any other Government agency. Also, if a particular brand name is not mentioned, this does not mean or imply that the product is unsatisfactory.

Like all medications, NSAIDs can have side effects. The list of possible adverse effects is long, but major problems are few. The intestinal tract heads the list with nausea, abdominal pain, vomiting, and diarrhea. Changes in liver function frequently occur in children (but not in adults) who use aspirin. Changes in liver function are rare in children using the other NSAIDs. Questions about the appropriate use of NSAIDs should be directed toward your health care provider or pharmacist.

Though not an NSAID, another commonly used OTC medication, acetaminophen (Tylenol), may relieve pain. It has no effect on inflammation, however.

Immobilization

Immobilization is a common treatment for sports injuries that may be done immediately by a trainer or paramedic. Immobilization involves reducing movement in the area to prevent further damage. By enabling the blood supply to flow more directly to the injury (or the site of surgery to repair damage from an injury), immobilization reduces pain, swelling, and muscle spasm and helps the healing process begin. Following are some devices used for immobilization:

Slings, to immobilize the upper body, including the arms and shoulders.

Splints and casts, to support and protect injured bones and soft tissue. Casts can be made from plaster or fiberglass. Splints can be custom made or ready made. Standard splints come in a variety of shapes and sizes and have Velcro straps that make them easy to put on and take off or adjust. Splints generally offer less support and protection than a cast, and therefore may not always be a treatment option.

Leg immobilizers, to keep the knee from bending after injury or surgery. Made from foam rubber covered with fabric, leg immobilizers enclose the entire leg, fastening with Velcro straps.

Surgery

In some cases, surgery is needed to repair torn connective tissues or to realign bones with compound fractures. The vast majority of sports injuries, however, do not require surgery.

Rehabilitation (Exercise)

A key part of rehabilitation from sports injuries is a graduated exercise program designed to return the injured body part to a normal level of function.

With most injuries, early mobilization—getting the part moving as soon as possible—will speed healing. Generally, early mobilization starts with gentle range-of-motion exercises and then moves on to stretching and strengthening exercise when you can without increasing pain. For example, if you have a sprained ankle, you may be able to work on range of motion for the first day or two after the sprain by gently tracing letters with your big toe. Once your range of motion is fairly good, you can start doing gentle stretching and strengthening exercises. When you are ready, weights may be added to your exercise routine to further strengthen the injured area. The key is to avoid movement that causes pain.

As damaged tissue heals, scar tissue forms, which shrinks and brings torn or separated tissues back together. As a result, the injury site becomes tight or stiff, and damaged tissues are at risk of reinjury. That's why stretching and strengthening exercises are so important. You should continue to stretch the muscles daily and as the first part of your warmup before exercising.

When planning your rehabilitation program with a health care professional, remember that progression is the key principle. Start with just a few exercises, do them often, and then gradually increase how much you do. A complete rehabilitation program should include exercises for flexibility, endurance, and strength; instruction in balance and proper body mechanics related to the sport; and a planned return to full participation.

Throughout the rehabilitation process, avoid painful activities and concentrate on those exercises that will improve function in the injured part. Don't resume your sport until you are sure you can stretch the injured tissues without any pain, swelling, or restricted movement, and monitor any other symptoms. When you do return to your sport, start slowly and gradually build up to full participation. For more advice on how to prevent injuries as you return to active exercise, see the "Tips for Preventing Injury" box.

Rest

Although it is important to get moving as soon as possible, you must also take time to rest following an injury. All injuries need time to heal; proper rest will help the process. Your health care professional can guide you regarding the proper balance between rest and rehabilitation.

Other Therapies

Other therapies commonly used in rehabilitating sports injuries include:

Electrostimulation: Mild electrical current provides pain relief by preventing nerve cells from sending pain impulses to the brain. Electrostimulation may also be used to decrease swelling, and to make muscles in immobilized limbs contract, thus preventing muscle atrophy and maintaining or increasing muscle strength.

Cold/cryotherapy: Ice packs reduce inflammation by constricting blood vessels and limiting blood flow to the injured tissues. Cryotherapy eases pain by numbing the injured area. It is generally used for only the first 48 hours after injury.

Heat/thermotherapy: Heat, in the form of hot compresses, heat lamps, or heating pads, causes the blood vessels to dilate and increase blood flow to the injury site. Increased blood flow aids the healing process by removing cell debris from damaged tissues and carrying healing nutrients to the injury site. Heat also helps to reduce pain. It should not be applied within the first 48 hours after an injury.

Ultrasound: High-frequency sound waves produce deep heat that is applied directly to an injured area. Ultrasound stimulates blood flow to promote healing.

Massage: Manual pressing, rubbing, and manipulation soothe tense muscles and increase blood flow to the injury site.

Most of these therapies are administered or supervised by a licensed health care professional.

Who Is at Greatest Risk for Sports Injuries?

If a professional athlete dislocates a joint or tears a ligament, it makes the news. But anyone who plays sports can be injured. Three groups—children and adolescents, middle-aged athletes, and women—are particularly vulnerable.

Children and Adolescents

Although playing sports can improve children's fitness, self-esteem, coordination, and self-discipline, it can also put them at risk for sports injuries: some minor, some serious, and still others that may result in lifelong medical problems.

Young athletes are not small adults. Their bones, muscles, tendons, and ligaments are still growing and that makes them more prone to injury. Growth plates—the areas of developing cartilage where bone growth occurs in growing children—are weaker than the nearby ligaments and tendons. As a result, what is often a bruise or sprain in an adult can be a potentially serious growth-plate injury in a child. Also, a trauma that would tear a muscle or ligament in an adult would be far more likely to break a child's bone.

Because young athletes of the same age can differ greatly in size and physical maturity, some may try to perform at levels beyond their ability to keep up with their peers.

Contact sports have inherent dangers that put young athletes at special risk for severe injuries. Even with rigorous training and proper safety equipment, youngsters are still at risk for severe injuries to the neck, spinal cord, and growth plates. Evaluating potential sports injuries on the field in very young children can involve its own special issues for concerned parents and coaches. Some helpful hints are presented in the appendix.

Adult Athletes

More adults than ever are participating in sports. Many factors contribute to sports injuries as the body grows older. The main one is that adults may not be as agile and resilient as they were when they were younger. It is also possible that some injuries occur when a person tries to move from inactive to a more active lifestyle too quickly.

Women

More women of all ages are participating in sports than ever before. In women's sports, the action is now faster and more aggressive and powerful than in the past. As a result, women are sustaining many more injuries, and the injuries tend to be sport specific.

Female athletes have higher injury rates than men in many sports, particularly basketball, soccer, alpine skiing, volleyball, and gymnastics. Female college basketball players are about six times more likely to suffer a tear of the knee's anterior cruciate ligament (ACL) than men are, according to a study of 11,780 high school and college players. Information on injuries collected since 1982 by the National Collegiate Athletic Association shows that female basketball and soccer players have a much higher incidence of ACL injuries than their male counterparts.

Previous assumptions that methods of training, risks of participation, and effects of exercise are the same for men and women are being challenged. Scientists are working to understand the gender differences in sports injuries.

Although poor conditioning has not been related to an increased incidence of ACL injuries specifically, it has been associated with an increase in injuries in general. For most American women, the basic level of conditioning is much lower than that of men. Studies at the U.S. Naval Academy revealed that overuse injuries were more frequent in women; however, as women became used to the rigors of training, the injury rates for men and women became similar.

Aside from conditioning level, other possible factors in women's sports injuries include structural difference of the knee and thigh muscles, fluctuating estrogen levels caused by menstruation, the fit of athletic shoes, and the way players jump, land, and twist. Also, "the female triad," a combination of disordered eating, curtailed menstruation (amenorrhea), and loss of bone mass (osteoporosis), is increasingly more common in female athletes in some sports. Its true prevalence is unknown, but it appears to be greater in athletes, adolescents, and young adults, especially in people who are perfectionists and overachievers.

Scientists trying to better understand sports injuries in women met in June 1999 for a workshop sponsored jointly by the National Institute of Arthritis and Musculoskeletal and Skin Diseases and the American Academy of Orthopaedic Surgeons. The workshop proceedings were published in a book titled Women's Health in Sports & Exercise, edited by William Garrett, M.D., Ph.D., and Gayle Lester, Ph.D. The book may be purchased from the American Academy of Orthopaedic Surgeons.

What Can Groups at High Risk Do to Prevent Sports Injuries?

Anyone who exercises is potentially at risk for a sports injury and should follow the injury prevention tips. But additional measures can be taken by groups at higher risk of injury.

Children

Preventing injuries in children is a team effort, requiring the support of parents, coaches, and the kids themselves. Here's what each should do to reduce injury risk.

What parents and coaches can do:

Try to group youngsters according to skill level and size, not by chronological age, particularly during contact sports. If this is not practical, modify the sport to accommodate the needs of children with varying skill levels.

Match the child to the sport, and don't push the child too hard into an activity that she or he may not like or be physically capable of doing.

Try to find sports programs where certified athletic trainers are present. These people, in addition to health care professionals, are trained to prevent, recognize, and give immediate care to sports injuries.

See that all children get a preseason physical exam.

Don't let (or insist that) a child play when injured. No child (or adult) should ever be allowed to work through the pain.

Get the child medical attention if needed. A child who develops any symptom that persists or that affects athletic performance should be examined by a health care professional. Other clues that a child needs to see a health professional include inability to play following a sudden injury, visible abnormality of the arms and legs, and severe pain that prevents the use of an arm or leg.

Provide a safe environment for sports. A poor playing field, unsafe gym sets, unsecured soccer goals, etc., can cause serious injury to children.

What children can do:

Be in proper condition to play the sport. Get a preseason physical exam.

Follow the rules of the game.

Wear appropriate protective gear.

Know how to use athletic equipment.

Avoid playing when very tired or in pain.

Make warmups and cooldowns part of your routine. Warmup exercises, such as stretching or light jogging, can help minimize the chances of muscle strain or other soft tissue injury. They also make the body's tissues warmer and more flexible. Cooldown exercises loosen the muscles that have tightened during exercise.

TIPS FOR PREVENTING INJURY

Whether you've never had a sports injury and you're trying to keep it that way or you've had an injury and don't want another, the following tips can help.

- Avoid bending knees past 90 degrees when doing half knee bends.
- Avoid twisting knees by keeping feet as flat as possible during stretches.
- When jumping, land with your knees bent.
- Do warmup exercises not just before vigorous activities like running, but also before less vigorous ones such as golf.
- Don't overdo.

Do warmup stretches before activity. Stretch the Achilles tendon, hamstring, and quadriceps areas and hold the positions. Don't bounce.

Cool down following vigorous sports. For example, after a race, walk or walk/jog for five minutes so your pulse comes down gradually.

Wear properly fitting shoes that provide shock absorption and stability.

Use the softest exercise surface available, and avoid running on hard surfaces like asphalt and concrete. Run on flat surfaces. Running uphill may increase the stress on the Achilles tendon and the leg itself.

Adult Athletes

To prevent injuries, adult athletes should take the following precautions:

- Don't be a "weekend warrior," packing a week's worth of activity into a day or two. Try to maintain a moderate level of activity throughout the week.

- Learn to do your sport right. Using proper form can reduce your risk of "overuse" injuries such as tendinitis and stress fractures.
- Remember safety gear. Depending on the sport, this may mean knee or wrist pads or a helmet.
- Accept your body's limits. You may not be able to perform at the same level you did 10 or 20 years ago. Modify activities as necessary.
- Increase your exercise level gradually.
- Strive for a total body workout of cardiovascular, strength training, and flexibility exercises. Cross-training reduces injury while promoting total fitness.

Women

Increased emphasis on muscle strength and conditioning should be a priority for all women. Women should also be encouraged to maintain a normal body weight and avoid excessive exercise that affects the menstrual cycle. In addition, women should follow precautions listed above for other groups.

What Are Some Recent Advances in Treating Sports Injuries?

Today, the outlook for an injured athlete is far more optimistic than in the past. Sports medicine has developed some near-miraculous ways to help athletes heal and, in most cases, return to sports. Following are some procedures that have greatly advanced the treatment of sports injuries:

Arthroscopy

Most doctors agree that the single most important

advance in sports medicine has been the development of arthroscopic surgery, or arthroscopy. Arthroscopy s a small fiberoptic scope inserted through a small inc in the skin to see inside a joint. It is primari diagnostic tool, allowing surgeons to view joint probl without major surgery. Depending on the probl found, surgeons may use small tools inserted through additional incisions to repair the damage, such as a torn meniscus or a torn ligament that fails to heal naturally. Using arthroscopy, for example, a surgeon may reattach the torn ends of a ligament or reconstruct the ligament by using a piece (graft) of healthy ligament from the patient or from a cadaver.

Because arthroscopy uses tiny incisions, it results in less trauma, swelling, and scar tissue than conventional surgery, which in turn decreases hospitalization and rehabilitation times. Problems can be diagnosed earlier and treated without serious health risks or more invasive procedures. Furthermore, because injuries are often addressed at an earlier stage, operations are more likely to be successful.

Tissue Engineering

When joint cartilage is damaged by an injury, it doesn't heal on its own the way other tissues do. In recent years, however, the field of sports medicine and orthopaedic surgery has begun to develop techniques such as transplantation of one's own healthy cartilage or cells to improve healing. At present, this technique is used for small cartilage defects. Questions remain about its usefulness and cost.

Targeted Pain Relief

For people with painful sports injuries, new pain-killing medicated patches can be applied directly to the injury site. The patch is an effective method of delivering pain relief, especially for many people who prefer to put their pain medication exactly where it's needed rather than throughout their entire system.

What Advances Might We Expect in the Future?

Recent advances in treating sports injuries are likely to be just the beginning. Watch for developments in these areas in the not-too-distant future:

The need for surgery may decline as improved rehabilitation techniques lead to a more "natural" progression to recovery for more musculoskeletal injuries.

Technical advances and new imaging methods will lead to better ways to diagnose and treat injuries.

Scientists will gain a better understanding of the role of nutrition in inflammation and healing. Such knowledge could lead to improvements in treatment.

Tissue engineering will become more commonplace. Studies of musculoskeletal tissue engineering are yielding promising results.

INJURIES PREVENTION

To prevent injuries it is necessary to have information about the factors that contribute to their occurrence. With this information we may understand the options for prevention. Effective injury prevention requires a multifaceted, multidisciplinary approach. Up to 50 percent of youth sports injuries are preventable, and parents and coaches can reduce injuries in young athletes by 80 percent if they follow some simple tips:

Warm up. Before you begin the physical workout,

warm-up your muscles for 10 minutes with light exercise.

Don't overdo it. Overexertion is the primary cause of injuries in adolescents.

Try variety. Your child shouldn't focus on just one sport. They need to develop strength everywhere.

Pump iron later. Hold off on weight training until it's appropriate. Children can't develop strength with weights until puberty and they need to be supervised when they do start using weights.

Build stronger girls. Because they lack testosterone, girls are more susceptible to injury. Because of that, girls need to focus on strength-training more than boys.

Focus on fitness. Fitness training should be included in all practices.

Listen to pain. Young athletes should not be encouraged to push through pain.

3

Arthrology

Arthrology is the science concerned with the anatomy, function, dysfunction and treatment of joints. Arthrology is a specialized area of anatomy that deals with the study and description of joints or articulations. By definition a joint or articulation exists where two or more skeletal components, whether bone or cartilage, come together or meet. For the athletic trainer the practical importance of acquiring a basic understanding of arthrology cannot be overemphasized. This information is important is understanding how joints normally function and in providing a basis for understanding the nature of joint injuries. Athletes are almost universally characterized by an ability to execute complex, highly coordinated, and purposeful movements. Without joints between bones and controlled and graceful movement of the athlete would be impossible; the body would be a rigid, immobile hulk. Simply stated, it is the existence of joints between bones that makes movement of body parts possible.

CLASSIFICATION OF JOINTS

Joints are classified into three major groups or types using either structural features or potential for movement as distinguishing criteria. For the athletic trainer, a system of joint classification using degree of movement is clearly the more functional and appropriate method.

On the basis, three joints classes can be identified: synarthroses, amphiarthroses, and diarthroses. If structural criteria are used for classification, these three joint classes are called, in the same order, fibrous, cartilaginous, and synovial.

Amphiarthroses

Slightly movable joints, or amphiarthroses, have a pad of either hyaline or fibrocartilage located between adjoining bony surface. There are two types of amphiarthrotic joints.

Sychrondrosis

In this type of joint in pad of hyaline cartilage joins one bone to another. Examples of synchondroses are the joints between rib pairs through to 'and the sternum.

Symphysis

Symphyses are articulations, generally located in the midline of the body, that have a pad of fibrocartilage between opposing bone surfaces. The pubic symphysis, the midline joint between the two hipbones in front is an example of this type of joint.

Synarthroses

There are three basic types of synarthrotic, or immovable, joints.

Syndesmosis

This type of synarthrotic joint is characterized by the presence of a dense fibrous membrane that binds the articular bone surfaces very closely and tightly to each other. Ligaments play an important role in restriction of movement in these joints. The articulation between the distal ends of the tribia and fibula is a good example of a syndesmosis.

Gomphosis

By definition a gomphosis is a synarthrotic or fibrous joint in which a conical peg or projection fits into a socket. Articulations between the roots of the teeth and sockets of the jaw bones are the only examples of this type of joint in the body. The fibrous type of membrane found between the root of the tooth and its socket is called the peridental membrane. Successful replacement of teeth that have been knocked out as a result of injury is possible if this membrane remains relatively undamaged.

Suture

True sutures are found only in the skull. As a group, sutures are not characterized by the substantial fibrous membranes or dense ligaments seen in syndesmoses. Instead, the adjoining bone margins are united into rigid, immovable joints by a series of jagged, interlocking processes. The sagittal suture between the two parietal bones of the skull is a good example of this joint type.

Diarthroses

Diarthrotic joints are often called synovial joints because they are characterized by the presence of a closed cavity, called the synovial or joint cavity, between the bones. As a group, the diarthrotic or synovial joints include by far by majority of the body's articulations. Because they are the most mobile of the three types of joints, they are functionally the most important. They also have the most complex structure and are most vulnerable to athletic injuries.

Synovial membrane

The deep, or cellular, layer of the joint capsule forms

the moist and slippery synovial membrane. It lines the joint space between opposing bones and attaches to the margins of the articular cartilage. Functionally, the synovial membrane secretes synovial fluid, or synovia, which serves to lubricate the joint and provide nourishment for the articular cartilage. The term "synovial" is form the Latin word meaning "with egg" because it resembles egg white in consistency and appearance. Synovial fluid will vary in amount from less than 0.1 ml to over 3.0 ml in different joints of the body. Quantity depends on both joint size and potential for movement.

Fibrous joint capsule

In movable joints a tough but flexible sleeve like structure called the joint capsule helps to hold the articulating bones together. The capsule encloses a space or cleft that exists between the opposing bone surfaces. The joint capsule consists of two layers: a tough, fibrous, outer layer called the fibrous capsule of the joint and a more cellular inner layer called the synovial membrane. Fibres in the outer layer of the joint capsule run in different directions to form a dense tubular structure that connects the periosteal membrane of one bone in the joint to that of the other.

The resulting fibrous layer of the capsule has great tensile strength that completely encases the ends of the bones and binds them to each other. This structure is uniquely constructed to resist shearing forces that would otherwise result in dislocation of opposing bone surfaces at the joint. The term "subluxation" is sometimes used to describe partial dislocations that occur if the capsule is stretched but not torn. At points of recurring stress in the capsule, fibres may become oriented in definite parallel bands to form inracapsular ligaments. These structures provide additional stability and help bind the bones together.

Articular Cartilage

The presence of specialized type of articular cartilage was included as one of six anatomic features common to long bones as a group. Articular, or hyaline, cartilage is a unique type of connective tissue. It consists of specialized cells called chondrocytes and a firm, gel like intercellular matrix. Very few fibres are present in hyaline cartilage and that the chondrocytes reside in little spaces called lacunae.

The intercellular matrix that surrounds the chondrocytes is similar to a fairly firm, smooth, plastic and, if kept lubricated, is superbly adapted for coating the articulating ends of bones in movable joints. Tough collagenous fibres anchor articular cartilage to the underlying bone and adjacent periosteal membrane. It is important to note that no blood vessels penetrate the gel like matrix of hyaline cartilage. It is said to be avanscular. For cells in cartilage tissue to survive without a direct blood supply, nutrients and oxygen must pass through the matrix bed by diffusion from synovial fluid. Diffusion over such distances is a slow and generally inefficient way to transfer nutrients to cells.

Indeed, in tissues other than cartilage it is not possible to sustain cell life if the normal blood supply is cut off. It is the unique diffusion mechanism of nutrient transfer in cartilage, however, that explains how bits of this tissue that detach from articulating bone surfaces by injury not only survive but also grow and increase in size. These small but sometimes troublesome bits of cartilage derive their nutrients by diffusion from the synovial fluid in the joint space. In addition to the thin layer of hyaline cartilage that covers the articulating bone surfaces in movable joints, pads of fibrocartilage may lie between the bones and divide the joint cavity.

These pads of fibrocartilage are called articular discs, or menisci. They provide an additional "cushion" between the articulating ends of the bones and help stabilize the joint. Fibrocartilage, as the name implies, contains a large number of collagenous fivers embedded in the matrix than is typical of hyaline.

The direct blood supply to fibrocartilage is little better, however, than that of the hyaline variety. Torn or damaged fibrocartilage in a joint quite often does not heal properly and must be removed by surgery. In most instances, only the damaged portion must be removed, thus saving as much of the structure as possible.

Types of Diarthroses

Diarthrotic joints are grouped or subdivided on the basis of :

1. The kind of movement each joint is capable of performing,

2. The shape of the surfaces of the adjacent articulating bones.

Uniaxial joints. Uniaxial joints permit movement in only one plane and around a single axis. There are two types of uniaxial joints: hinge and pivot.

Hinge joints such as the elbow permit movement only about one axis, which passes through the joint from side to side. Only flexion and extension occur in hinge joints. Because they allow movement in only one plane, hinge joints are those most often involved in athletic injuries. Typically, the single axis of pivot joints is vertical.

In this type of uniaxial joint, movement is limited to rotation. In pivot joints a type of bony ring on one bone rotates around a pivot point on another bone. For example, the first cervical vertebra, or atlas, acts as a bony ring that rotates around a conical pivot process called the dens on the second cervical vertebra, or axis. This joint permits you to turn your head from side to side.

Biaximal joints. In biaximal joints, movement occurs in two planes and around two axes that are the right angles to each other. Flexion and extension are allowed around one axis and abduction and adduction around the second axis. There are two types of biaximal joints: saddle and condyloid.

The articular surface of one bone in a saddle joint is concave in one direction and convex in the other, whereas the articular surface of the remaining bone is exactly the opposite. The opposing saddle-shaped surfaces fit neatly together, permitting flexion and extension around one axis and abduction and adduction around the other. The carpometacarpal joint at the base of the thumb is the only saddle joint in the body. Articulation occurs between the proximal end of the metacarpal bone of the thumb and the carpal bone named the trapezium.

Condyloid joints are those in which an oval condyle fits into an elliptic socket or cavity. This type of articular surface permits angular movement in two planes, but not axial rotation.

In short, it permits biaximal movement. The radius joins the carpal bones by means of a condyloid joint. Movements in the frontal plane are called radical and ulnar flexion. Radial flexion is movement at the wrist of the thumb side of the hand toward the forearm. Ulmar flexion is movement at the wrist of the little finger side of the hand toward the forearm.

Multiaxial joints. Multiaxial joints have two or more axes of rotation and permit movement in three or more planes. There are two types of multiaxial joints: ball-and-socket and gliding.

Ball-and-socket joints are those in which a ball shaped head of one bone fits into a concave socket or depression of another bone. Of all the joints in our bodies, ball-and-socket joints permit the widest and freest range of movements in almost any direction or place. Movements in this type of joint include flexion, extension, abduction, adduction, rotation, and circumduction. Examples are the shoulder and hip joints.

Gliding joints are numerous and almost always small. Articular surfaces in these joints are either flat, nearly flat, or slightly curved. They include most of the joints between both the carpal and tarsal bones and also all the joints between the articular processes of the vertebrae. These joints allow only the simplest kind of slight displacement motion between their articular surfaces. Gliding movements occur in all planes.

Range and type of movement in diarthroses

Range of motion

Diarthrotic or synovial, joints are often referred to as "freely movable joints". Such as description, of course, applies only to the normal direction and range of motion available at any particular joint.

Even for the most supple athlete there are distinct and necessary limitations to joint mobility. The normal type and range of join movements are influenced primarily by four factors:

1. The number, type of attachment and tautness of ligaments;

2. The shape of the articular or join surfaces;

3. The restraining effects of the joint capsule, and

4. The effect of muscles that may act as fixators to stabilize the joint. In addition, there is also frequent and sometimes considerable variation in the range of movement among individuals.

Repeated observations of ROM in both active and passive movements at a joint will prove helpful in visualizing the underlying anatomy. In active movements the athlete voluntarily moves a joint or body part through its pain-free ROM and in passive movements the athletic trainer moves the part with the muscles relaxed.

Normally, both active and passive range of motion manoeuvres should be about equal.

Types of Movement

Although we have the ability to perform a single movement at a single joint at one time, most coordinated types of body activity occur only as a result of simultaneous or successive movements at many joints. Articulating bones in synovial joints, acting in conjunction with other joints, are capable of moving in many directions, along different axes of rotation, and through different planes of reference in the body.

The various types of combines joint movements that occur as a result of such activity can be categorized or grouped as follows:

1. angular if there is a change in the angle between bones,

2. rotation and circumduction if there is movement of a bone around its own axis,

3. gliding if the only movement produced is simple displacement between articulating surfaces, and

4. special if the movement produced is so unique that it must be described individually.

Angular movements

Flexion decreases the size of the angle between the anterior or posterior surfaces of articulated bones. An exception to this definition is the shoulder joint. Shoulder flexion occurs as the arm is elevated forward in the sagittal plane. Flexing movements are bending or folding movements. Bending the head forward on the chest, for example, is flexion of the joint between the occipital bone at the base of the skull and the atlas, or first cervical vertebra. Bending the elbow, as when the forearm bends back on the arm, is another example of flexion.

Abduction is movement of a body part or extremity away from the midline or centre of the body. An example of abduction is movement of the arm away from the body in the frontal plane.

Horizontal abduction is movement of the upper limb through the transverse plane at shoulder level away from the midline of the body.

Extension is the return from the flexed position and generally results in an increase of a joint angle. Whereas bending movements are flexion, straightening, or stretching movements are extension. Most major joints are in extension when a person restores an extremity or body part from a flexed position to the anatomic position. Continuation of extension beyond the anatomic position is called hyperextension. Extension of the head, for example, means to return it to the upright anatomic position from the flexed position; hyperextension of the head would result in its being stretched backward from the upright position.

Flexion and extension of the ankle joint are termed plantar and dorsal flexion. Plantar flexion is movement of the sole of the foot downward, such as standing on your toes. Dorsiflexion is movement of the top of the foot upward.

Adduction is the opposite of abduction. It moves the body part toward the midline or centre of the body. An example would be bringing the arms back to the sides of the body from the abducted position.

Horizontal adduction is movement of the upper limb through the transverse plane at shoulder level toward the midline of the body. In discussing abduction and adduction of the fingers and toes the plane of reference is not the midline of the body but an imaginary line drawn through the midline finger or second toe. Movement of the fingers or toes away from these imaginary reference lines results in "spreading" movements or abduction. Movement of the fingers or toes toward these imaginary reference lines results in adduction.

Rotation and Circumduction

Rotation is the pivoting of a bone on its own central or longitudinal axis, somewhat as a top turns on its axis. An example is holding your head in an upright position and turning it from one side to the other, as in saying no.

Circumduction is a composite movement that combines flexion, abduction, extension, and adduction. The result is rotational movement that causes the segment as a whole to describe a cone as it moves.

Gliding movements

Gliding is the simplest type of movement that can occur in movable joints and occurs to some degree in all of them. In some joints this type of slight relative displacement between adjoining bone surfaces is the only type of motion available. Gliding movements occur when one articulating bone surface in a joint moves over another, unaccompanied by angular or rotary movement. Movement between the carpal bones of the wrist is largely gliding in nature.

Special movements

Pronation describes the inward rotation or movement of the supinated forearm and hand, which causes the palm of the hand to face posteriorly. In pronation the radius crosses diagonally over the ulna in the forearm. The position of the hands when you do a push-up is an example of the hands and forearms in pronation.

In inversion the sole of the foot is turned inward and the inner margin of the foot is raised. This is the movement most commonly associated with a sprained ankle.

In eversion the foot is turned so that the sole faces outwards and its outer margin is raised. Inversion and eversion movements take place within the subtler and transverse tarsal joints.

Elevation results in upward movement, whereas depression is a lowering of a body part or return from an elevated position. These terms are used most commonly to describe movements of the mandible and shoulder girdle.

Supination takes place at the radioulnar joint. In the anatomic position the hands and forearms are already supinated. The radius and ulna of the forearm and parallel and that the palm of the hand faces anteriorly in the supinated position. A handball serve involves supinating the hand.

Protraction refers to motion that moves a part forward. Reaching for an object involves protraction of the shoulder girdle. This is also known as scapula abduction.

Retraction is the motion that returns a protracted body part to its original or usual position. Retraction is also known as scapular adduction.

Joint disorders - arthritis is the name given to inflammation of a joint. There are three types:

osteoarthritis - this is the most common type of arthritis affecting 90% of all arthritis sufferers. It is associated with deterioration of the articular cartilage which then leads to the formation of calcifications or bone spurs. These bone spurs irritate the articular capsule and cause pain. Little, if any, actual inflammation occurs. The articular cartilage deteriorates because of age, stress, and injury.

Rheumatoid arthritis - This is the most severely debilitating form of arthritis, but affects less than 10% of arthritis sufferers. It is considered an autoimmune disease and begins with immune system cells releasing chemicals which attack the joint tissues. Severe inflammation results in great pain. The inflamed tissues become infused with fibrous tissue causing great stiffness and this fibrous tissue may eventually ossify to form bony connections which render the joints immobilized and visibly misshapen. Pain relieving drugs and surgery, even joint replacement, are the treatments.

Gouty arthritis - the gout is a genetic disorder of the ability to metabolize uric acid. Uric acid is a product of the breakdown of certain nucleic acids. Most people convert it to urea for excretion. In these individuals uric acid crystals build up in the soft joint tissues and causes their inflammation and destruction. It is especially likely to affect the big toe. Anti-inflammatory drugs and dietary restrictions are the treatment.

4

Physical Fitness, Warm-Up and Limber-Down

MEANING OF PHYSICAL FITNESS

The term 'Fitness' are the aspects that lead individuals to happiness, Physical Education helps in developing those aspects. To work efficiently and in productive manner it is essential for any individual to keep himself/ herself physically fit. So that the same can work for wellness of mankind. Following this paragraph the given subject matter clears us about the term 'Physical Fitness and Wellness' .Now a days great emphasis is being given on good looking, healthy feeling and energetic approaches. To achieve the ideals regular physical exercises and knowledge about muscular movements is necessary. Present modern scenario demanding not much of physical effort by providing new technologies and efficient machinery. As fewer jobs now a day require physical exertion, it is very important to give some extra work to human body in a well recreational manner to recharge and fit our self. In the following section we will be analyzing general and basic instruction or information that is needed to maintain personal physical fitness and wellness.

PHYSICAL FITNESS

Physical fitness is the organic vagueness or the proper functioning of body systems so that individual can perform the daily routine tasks efficiently. It is the ability to perform daily activity, with energy left over for enjoying leisure-time activities and meeting emergency demands if any. It is the ability to endorse, to bear up, and to withstand stress to carry on in circumstances where an unfit person could not continue. Physical fitness indicates how much accurately a work is done by an individual and even after the workout how much of energy is stored in him/her to perform other needed activities in a well skilled manner. It is clear and obvious that after workout every individual gets fatigue, this applies to every physical fit person but one of the major difference in unfit and fit individual is the storage of energy for emergency and other normal activities even after fatigue, other major aspect in physical fitness is the fast recovery after getting tired. After fatigue work rest is necessary but the rest period must be of appropriate duration. Physical fitness is the continuation of daily routine work without Undue fatigue.

The below given Fatigue-Recovery cycle represents an average human beings physical fitness approaches. In this cycle this is shown clearly that every individual get-tired or feel fatigue after performing daily work out efficiently. But this fatigue must not lead to complete rest of individual and no more work after that. The fatigue after main workout cannot lead to stoppage of further task for any physical fit person. Storage of energy must be present to perform other needed activities or leisure time activities in an efficient and well manner. Apart From this capacity of performing main workout and other general activities, availability of appropriate energy must still be there to meet any emergency demands. The energy expenditure medium of an average individual is his/her main workout with other daily needed activities plus the emergency requirements (energy expenditure on emergency is situational and very rare) which definitely produce tiredness (Fatigue). After Fatigue proper rest is highly required and quick and total recovery from tiredness is again the indication of Physical fitness. A fit person also requires rest and the time needed for the rest determines the fitness level. If we take example of two individuals, they may require different time period of rest after performing same workout. Total recovery recharges individual to get ready for performing tasks again.

Physical Fitness gives us better look, pleasant feel and productive performance. Fitness is an individual quality that differs from individual to individual. Physical fitness involves the performance of our body systems like circulatory system, Muscular system etc. but the intellectual abilities, alertness, emotional stability etc also shown its affect on physical fitness. Psychological set up also having influences in physical fitness.

DEFINING PHYSICAL FITNESS:

"Physical fitness refers to the organic capacity of the individual to perform the normal task of daily living without undue tiredness or fatigue having reserves of strength and energy available to meet satisfactorily any emergency demands suddenly placed upon him."

—Nixon

"Physical Fitness is the ability of a person to do daily routine work without fatigue; moreover to participate in playful activity and still reserves enough capacity to meet any emergency."

—Webster

"Physical fitness is the state which characterizes the

degree to which the person is able to function. It implies the ability of each person to live most effectively with his potential. Ability to function depends upon physical, mental, emotional and social components of fitness, all of which are related to each other and mutually interdependent."

—Kirchner

"Physical Fitness is the successful adaptation to the stresses of one's life style."

—Krolc

IMPORTANCE OF PHYSICAL FITNESS

Physical fitness and wellness is not only the need of high performers in sports, rather every individual need physical fitness and wellness for a well balanced life Some importance of physical fitness and wellness are explained below:-

(1) Physiological Efficiency increases

a) Improved function of circulatory system- Heart's weight, volume and capacity increases. Resting heart rate decreases and stroke volume, which is the amount of blood plumbed by the left or right ventricle of the heart per beat, increases, which assist for good cardiac output. Due to increase in blood volume (which is mainly due to increase in blood plasma volume) and other given benefits function of heart increases.

b) Improved function of Respiratory system:

Long volume and capacity increases. Breathing frequency (number of breaths per minute) is decreased, this reduction increases respiratory efficiency. Increase Maximum minute ventilation (amount of air, inspires/

expires in one minute) increases the work efficiency. Venially efficiency of respiratory system assists physically fit person in some life threatening situations. Increase in tidal volume (amount of air inspired or expired per breath) and pulmonary effective diffusion (exchanges of gases taken place in the alveoli) increases the working capacity.

c) Increase function of Muscles- Thickness in individual muscle fiber (hypertrophy) and increased amount of proteins in the muscles of physically fit person enhances strength and muscular endurance. The working capacity also depends upon the presence of muscular energy. Glycogen is essential for energy production in the muscles, amount of glycogen store increases if individual is physically fit.

d) Effective Metabolism and catabolism occurs, oxidation of carbohydrate and fat increases and some other chemical changes increase energy, depending upon physical fitness and wellness of an individual.

e) Effectiveness increases as other system also like digestive system, immune system etc. improves. Glandular functions also improve which assists in balanced growth of child.

f) Standard body composition. Significant losses of relative and absolute fact of body increases fitness components mainly flexibility. Muscle mass increases significantly. Joints and other soft tissues (muscle tendon, ligaments) also get strengthen which also helps in preventing injuries.

g) Reduced cholesterol levels assists individual to be away from some diseases.

h) Physical fitness and wellness assists in

maintaining good posture.

2. Social efficiency increases:

a) Improved self-image- Healthy and well-balanced personality increases ones self/image. This improved self-image creates great self-respect in the personality.

b) Social adaptability- the behaviour of well being increases his/her social acceptance and one can manage easily in the society and in some way society feel glad on him/her.

c) Increased Role in society- Society is always ready to give every opportunity to those individuals who have all components of physical fitness and wellness.

d) Social recognition- A person who is socially acceptable and playing effective role in society will definitely get special recognition and status in society.

e) Other qualities like good character, discipline, loyalty, individual advancement increases as wellness increases in an individual.

3. Psychological and Mental efficiency increases-

a. Mental alertness sharpens the thinking ability and increases efficiency- As stimulation system increases the individual becomes more alert and sharp. The mental capacity of an individual increases so that same can act purposefully, think rationally and deal effectively with one's environment.

b. Stress Management- Good physical fitness and wellness increases the skill of stress Management. Control and managing stress is needed for success in every field, this helps individual to go happy and perform well.

c. Motivation-Components of physical fitness and wellness make individual more motivated. Motivation is force, which energizes an individual.

d. Physical fitness and wellness brings vice thoughts and feelings, which is always healthy for society and oneself. It helps in overcoming Aggression and anxiety. (Aggression is needed to some extent).

e. Personal Habits for betterment of self and society. Increases Habits like keeping oneself calm and active, living in hygienic atmosphere, creating healthy environment etc. will ensure good and productive workout.

Therefore, no doubt that physical fitness and wellness contributes a lot in gaining high performances and also reduces risk of major illness like diabeties, heart diseases or psychological defects like depression etc.

COMPONENTS OF PHYSICAL FITNESS AND AFFECTING FACTORS

Components of physical fitness can be said as products, which collectively constitute physical fitness and wellness. Each component is equally essential. These components are highly related to each other and therefore one component directly or indirectly influences the other. Presence of all components in good grade is essential. In other words a good performer needs to have every component and that too with effective ratio. For example, power and speed is as valuable for a thrower as muscular strength. Six components are given below:

1. Strength
2. Power
3. Speed

4. Agility
5. Endurance
6. lexibility

1. Strength:

Exertion of force against resistance.

Strength is the ability of muscles to overcome resistance. It is the ability to exert a force against a resistance. Type of strength needed for one kind of work may not be needed for other kind of work. For example 'power lifter' and a Runner both need different kind of strength. Strength is the capability of the muscles force that comes out by constriction to overcome. Therefore three types of strength as explained below:

a) Maximum strength - It is the force exerted in a single maximum contraction of muscle. Maximum strength is the force of greatest potential exerted by muscle to over come a resistance in a single maximum contraction. Activities requiring maximum strength mainly is weight/lifting, power/lifting etc.

b) Explosive Strength: Exertion of force by quick contraction of muscle is explosive strength. It is the ability to overcome a resistance with fast contractions. In the combination of speed and strength is power and explosive strength .It increase the ability to overcome resistance with a fast counteraction.

The combination of speed and strength is power and explosive strength actually is the combing of speed and strength. Therefore explosive strength can also be said as power, which is offcourse one of the main component of physical fitness, Activities involving forming or boarding essentially need explosive strength.

c) Strength Endurance- Exertion of force for long duration is strength Endurance. It is the ability to express over a longer period of time. It is quite apparent from the terminology that strength with endurance component. It is the ability to overcome resistance under fatigue (or longer duration). Activities of longer duration need this element of physical fitness.

2. Speed: Generally speaking speed is considered as The quickness Speed is the quick movements of limbs. Speed is a skill of performing movements of limbs at quicker rate. Speed is said as the basic component of physical fitness. Moving the limbs or muscles are quick as possible is very complex procedure, which is controlled by the brain and nervous system. Depending upon the demand of quickness of muscles speed can also be divided in Following aspects.

a) Maximum Speed- In this type of speed Maximum possible quickness of muscles is shown. The movement of limbs in the fastest way possible is maximum speed. Activities like sprints need maximum speed through the quick contraction of muscles so that quick movement of limbs can be possibly done.

b) Explosive strength-Power is also known as Explosive strength. Example is the starting phase of a sprinter. In this phase the athlete needs both components, (i) speed for quick movement of limbs and (ii) strength the start effectively by overcoming resistance and forceful forward movement. Power is the ability to exert maximum muscular force instantly in a explosive best of movement.

c) Speed Endurance- quickness of movement of limb for longer duration is speed endurance. It is a combination of two elements (i) speed and (ii)

Endurance. Medium distances running events is one of the example, that require this element of physical fitness.

3. Agility:

Quick explosive power movements in various directions are the agility of an individual. Performing any cutting movements or Game drills with application of power component is said to be exposing the component Agility. Agility is the ability to perform a series of explosive power movements in rapid succession in various directions. The movements performed in opposite direction in a successive way are actually for enhancing the agility of that performer. Specific activity zigzag running is mainly for the development of Agility. It is the ability of an individual to change directions quickly while moving. Agility is the capability of a person to change his/her body positions quickly with well-balanced movements. Ability to start quickly and abrupt stopping of movement and changing body positions are Agility.

4. Endurance:

Ability to perform maximum amount of work over an extended period of time is Endurance. It is the ability to sustain activity and to resist and fatigue. Endurance is also briefed as developed energy production system. This system is general can be briefed as Oxygen supplied to working muscles and proper utilization decides the capacity of performer. Therefore for good cardiovascular endurance proper and efficient functioning of circulatory and respiratory system is must .Activity wise Endurance is of four types.

i Aerobic Endurance/ All kind of activities with

oxygen require `Aerobic Endurance. Aerobic means with oxygen. These activities long from 2 minutes to 30 minutes (or more).

ii. Anaerobic Endurance- All kind of activities without oxygen in taking requires Anaerobic Endurance. Anaerobic means without oxygen. These activities some time are even of less than 10 sec. But can be extended up to 120 seconds.

iii. Speed Endurance/ quickness of movement of limb for longer duration is speed endurance.

iv. Strength Endurance- Exertion of force for long duration is strength Endurance.

5. Flexibility: Range of motion of joints is flexibility of an individual. It is the ability to moving joints in full range of motion. It is obvious that its because of muscles movement is performed, therefore flexibility is that quality of the muscles that enables the joints of the body to move easily through a complete range of movement. Flexibility determines the extent of extension and flexion of a joint. The type of joint determines the degree of flexibility. Flexibility is essential for good performance and it also presents performer from injuries.

i. Static flexibility. Performing flexibility in a stationary position is static flexibility. Static stretching exercises like long splitting, forward bending etc. are used for static flexibility.

ii. Dynamic flexibility- performing flexibility while in motion is dynamic flexibility. Movement stretching exercises like arm rotation, toe touching etc. are used for dynamic flexibility.

1. Active flexibility Exercises: In this method athlete perform flexible exercises by him self. This method

doesn't involve any help from other athlete/individual. It involves the active participation of the performer himself. Any self-performing flexibility exercise comes under this method.

2. Passive flexibility Exercises_ In this method athlete performs flexible exercises with the help of his partner. This method involves active participation of partner also, who helps the performer in gaining the maximum range of flexibility. This requires good understanding between the performer and his partner.

Apart from the above given basic components of physical fitness, which are also known as Elements of physical fitness, Co-ordination is some time also included in the list, coordination is some time also included in the list Coordination is the ability to integrate these six up given components so that effective movement can occur.

FACTORS AFFECTING PHYSICAL FITNESS:

Physical fitness is an individual quality that differs from person to person. This statement widens the affecting aspects. It can be said that almost any individual quality would affect physical fitness, like attitude of an individual, habits, liking or disliking of an individual can have its affects on physical fitness of that individual.

(i) PERSONAL HABITS - A person in habit of regular exercises, not necessarily specific exercises but if even a habit of general morning walk will definitely be having its affect on fitness. Habits of late night sleep, alcohol liking, over eating, etc can be big a hindrance to get oneself physically fit.

(ii) BALANCED DIET - In maintaining oneself

balanced diet is off course effective. To maintain a good level of physical fitness there must be good balance between energy intake and energy output. Over intake of calories than our body needs will put on more fat. Diet itself varies from individual to individual, depends on many factors like age, sex, type of physical training.

(iii) AGE - Human beings in different age groups run with different physiological and psychological characteristics. Many physical fitness components have direct relation with the physiological changes like strength element of in an infant and adult. The physical fitness mainly depends on the growth and development of muscles, bones, sensory system and other organs. As human become older his functional systems becomes weaker, which results in low fitness.

(iv) SEX - Up to 12 - 13 years of age, there is not much difference in body composition of boys and girls. There up to this age period both sex have almost same physical fitness level. But at maturity they become different significantly on various parameters. These physical, physiological and anthropometrical differences also affect the physical fitness of male and female.

(v) PSCHOLOGICAL ASPECTS - Factors like anxiety, attention and concentration, arousal and aggressiveness have its direct or indirect influence in fitness of an individual. Over showing of these factors are harmful and gain fitness but this does't mean these factors are not needed to get fitness and better performance. Anxiety aggressiveness etc to some extent are necessary for good performance. Attitude is also influential to large extent as every achievement depends on attitude towards the activity and liking and disliking creates interest in an individual to achieve good personality,. This assists individual to develop physical fitness. If a child says I like playing, it reflects his attitudes towards playing. Apart from anxiety, attention, concentration, aroosal, aggressiveness and attitudes. Mental imagery and motivation, interest etc are some other psychological factors which affect physical fitness and wellness.

(vi) REGULAR EXERCISES/WORKOUT - Regular workout keeps our body systems efficient level of physical fitness and wellness depends largely on regularity. The more regular one is in workout the more fit he will be their must be containing in practice.

(vii) INSTITUTIONAL CURRICULAR PROGRAMME- Fitness and wellness of child also depends on child's institution's curricular programme. This institution may be a family itself, educational institution, a state or friends circle.

(viii) HEREDITY - Human skeletal muscle can be classified into three different types based on biochemical characteristics of the individual muscle cells. The classification is:-

(a) Fast twist fibre - Leg muscles of sprinters are composed principally of fast twist fibers. (These muscle fibres contain small number of mitochondria but rich in glycogen, therefore F T fibres provide klarge anaerobic capacity).

(b) Slow twist fibre - Leg muscle of clime distance runners is composed principally of slow twist fibres. (These muscle fibres contain large number of mitochondria and rich in myoglobin, therefore ST fibres provide large aerobic capacity).

(c) Intermediate fibres - These are not a single fibre type because some intermediate fibers have biochemical and contract property similar to FT fibers while other intermediate fibres have biochemical and contractile property similar to ST fibers.

(ix) SYSTEMATIC EXERCISES - Systematic and scientific training is essential to get productive results. Training must be planned scientifically and then must be followed systematically. Proper loading, over loading, proper rest and recreational processes are essential factors to gain and maintain fitness.

(ix) BODY COMPOSITION AND BODY POSTURE- For an individual with excessive fat its hard to maintain some component of fitness in good grade like flexibility, endurance etc. In same way an individual with postural defects like kyphosis, knock knee, scoliosis etc its hard to perform effectively some exercises which may resist him to gain fitness in good grade.

(x) ENVIRONMENT AND PROFESSIONAL DEMAND- Any individual is highly influenced by his surrounding environment and by profession demands on him. Now a day's society prefers parties more than any collective playing, this affects the fitness level of society member. Similarly long sittings for office work lead to bad posture, which affect ones fitness level. Environmental factors like dehydration, acclimatization, humidity etc also affects the components of physical fitness.

(xi) GRADUAL PROGRESSION OF LOAD: Gradual progression of load is highly required for the achievement of high fitness level. Abrupt progression or injury of muscles. The approach should be step by step, well planned and maintained. Gradual progressive development helps in gaining better fitness level. Maintenance and adoption of land must be taken into consideration before approaching for more lead.

PRINCIPLES OF PHYSICAL FITNESS DEVELOPMENT

The basic principles to develop physical fitness are given below:

(i) PRINCIPLE OF SPECIFICITY, SCIENTIFIC AND SYSTEMATIC WORKOUT

Specificity is required to concentrate on every component of fitness separately. Methods of specificity are required to meet the specific demands. As all components are well related and even depended on one or the other components, this methodology is very useful. Scientific way to workout/training is the need of the hour. Programmes for the development of physical fitness must be planned scientifically and systematically. Highly advanced scientific processes will assist individual to develop components systematically and in a progressive way. Proper warming up and cooling down is best example of scientific training.

(ii) PRINCIPLE OF INDIVIDUALITY:

A different principle to be followed for different individuals, as fitness is an individual quality. Any mean or method effective for one person may not be good enough for other. Processes for the development of physical fitness should be prepared and planned as per individual's own ability. Age and sex differences itself proves the principles accuracy. Height, ability, heredity, environment are also the aspects to be kept in mind while preparing programmes for physical fitness.

(iii) PRINCIPLE OF CONTINUITY:

Elements of physical fitness require continues effort. To develop components become more challenging if continuity is lost. The training effect will reverse itself if there is no continuity, non existence of continuity in programmes may lead to now fitness level, Principle of continuity must not be confused with principle of rest and principle of overloading. Sometimes training programme needs deliberate breaks. Regular workout keeps our body systems efficient level of physical fitness depends largely on regularity/continuity.

(iv) PRINCIPLE OF OVERLOAD OR PRINCIPLE OF ADAPTATION OF LOAD:

Any improvement in fitness requires an increased training load so that the individual's state of fitness can be challenged. Scientific increase in load increases the capacity. Any kind of increase on load shall only be planned after proper adaptation of load by the individual. Overloading may cause reduction in fitness and some time severe other complication also. Gradual progression of load is highly required for the achievement of high fitness level. Abrupt load may also lead to over fatigue or injury of muscles.

(v) PRINCIPLE OF APPROPRIATE REST AND RECOVERY:

Appropriate rest and recovery is required to recharge oneself, so that same can continue his workout to develop fitness. Continuation of workout even under fatigue may lead to injuries and other complications. To recreate energy system proper rest and recovery for fatigue or any kind of injuries is essentially required. Recovery or rest period must be systematically planned and followed on. Rest period depends upon the level of training also. High intensity work may need more rest period than low intensity. Lengthy rest period depends upon the fitness level of athlete

(vi) PRINCIPLE OF ACTIVE PARTICIPATION.

Individual must be actively involved in this process by his/her own choice. Lack of active participation lead to severe complications like injuries, psychological defects etc. Interest and mental preparedness are the main aspect of this principle. Therefore the training programmes planned must be interesting and alive in nature. Activeness increases the working efficiency and make athlete more safety and confidential motivational.

(vii) Principle of safety and preventive measures- Work out done with all its safety and preventive measures will be more productive then working with unsafe or unproductive plan. This principle also increases the working efficiency and more concentration can be paid in fitness programmes. For achieving good performance and fitness level by any athlete is essential to be fearless and confident. Proper safety steps and preventive measures help in developing principal of fitness.

(vii) PSYCHOLOGICAL FEED BACK-

Motivation, good spirit presence of mind, Attention and concentration etc. Group dynamics psychological feedback definitely enhances working capacity of an individual, which ultimately helps in improving fitness components. Psychological feedback should be provided in a positive manner. Fitness of an individual also depends upon the psychological aspects of the same individual and valuable for the development of fitness level of athlete as other.

WARM-UP AND LIMBER-DOWN

WARMING UP-

Warming up is pre-exercise workout. It is a

preparation for the activity; this preparation includes physiological and psychological aspects. Warm/up is accomplished of general as well as specific body movements in order to make all body systems ready for the activity.

The terminology warm/up is actually applied because warming/up, warms or increases the body core temperature, which enhances physiological efficiency. Psychology is also considered as essential base of warming/up. In real terms warm/up have its direct influence in physiological systems but if an individual has not interest to do activity, nothing can be learned by him/her, therefore psychological preparation is considered as essential base of warm-up.

Type of Warming-up.

1. Physiological warming/up- preparation of body systems for the main work out is physiological warming-up. This includes the physical exercises and different tasks performed physically. Variation in body temperature, more range of motion, improved Co-ordination, better blood circulation etc. is result of physiological warming- up, and there are two types of physiological warming- up.

a) General warming-up

b) Specific Warming Up.

a) General warming up: It covers general physical movements, which are required almost before every Game and sport. It aims for preparing athlete to perform basic movements and then only athlete can approach for specific movements. Physical exercises in general warming up are general in nature. Jogging simple striding, general stretching exercises etc. are the exercises, which mainly performed in it. General warning- up target for major muscle groups and joints.

b) Specific warming - up-It covers those kind of exercise which mainly prepares athletic for performing some specific movement. It aims to perform that movement which athlete has to perform in main activity. Unlike exercise of general warming up. Have exercises are differ sport to sport. Physical exercises in it are specific in nature. Dummy actions, exercises perfecting skills is specific warming- up specific warming - up target for specific muscle group.

2. Psychological warming -up- mental preparation for the work our is psychological warming athletic psychologically accepting the hard work him / her for better performance with all needed feedback which leads for concentration needed behaviour etc, In high level sports competitions much depends on psychological preparation.

Guidelines of Proper Warming-Up

Duration of warming up- It depends on many factors. It also differ form individual to individual. Training period, climate, type of activity etc. are the depending factors, the duration must be between 12 to 30 minutes, but can be extended for more duration if necessary.

METHODS OF WARMING UP

Warming up are:

1. Active warming up- It involves self/performed workout. Active way of warming up is physically self-involved participation in workout. This method brings physiological changes by general and specific exercises.
1. Active Warming up-

2. Passive Warming up- This method of warming up involved supportive or external way of exercises. Instead of physical self-involved participation, it`is done by external sources .It bring physiological changes by external sources such as steam bath, massage etc.

Warming up

SEQUENCE OF WARMING- UP AND PROPER PLANNING.

Warm up must be well planned and do sequentially, unsequencial and unplanned warm- up may result in unskillful performance or injuries . This also affect psychological aspects (like low motivation, less concentration etc). Exercises are preferably from top to bottom and bottom to top.

4. Degree of Difficulty:

General warm up must start with very low degree of difficulty and progression must be acdceptable to athlete. Therefore initially simple fogging followed by stretching and simple exercises for large muscles can be performed.

5. Age, sex, fitness and level of performance of an athlete must be taken into consideration.

IMPORTANCE OF WARMING UP

1. It increases body temperature that makes body systems more efficient and ready to accept load come from activity.

2. Second wind comes at the earliest possible.

3. It improves Neuro Muscular co-ordination that assists athlete to perform with increased agility, good reaction time, more flexibility.

4. Physiological benefits like increased muscle and

ligaments flexibility during Warming up reduces the chances of injuries.

5. It improves or controls psychological aspects that helps in reduction of tension and gain more concentration and confidence. The psychological aspects assist in gaining physiological advantages through the factors like controlled blood pressure, prepared heart rate etc.

6. Warming up therefore leads to better skill and better overall performance reason being.

LIMBERING DOWN

Limbering down is past exercise workout. In limbering down the intensity of activity done is lowered. It mainly includesstretching and other relaxative exercises. Slow jogging with deep breathing exercises etc.

The terminology 'Limbering down' is the cooling of core body temperature, which brings the physiological systems as efficient as needed in normal working conditions. Limbering down aims for regaining normal body temperature slowly (because abrupt change in body temperature may lead to harmful effects).

Types of Limbering Down:

1. Physiological Limbering down - Regaining the normal functioning of physiological systems back to average heart beat of 50-70 per minute) after the main workout is physiological limbering-down. This too includes the physical exercises and different tasks performed physically. Stretching exercises are preferable.

2. Psychological Limbering down - While doing main

activity or competition an athlete psychology is totally different, compared to psychology of the same athlete is in its normal social life. Psychological regaining the normal functioning (no aggressiveness) is the aim of it. Psychological limbering down is also preferable because while performing athlete can also think of mistakes done in main activity. Performing "SAWA ASSAN' is the best example of this or simply closing eyes and recollecting the mistakes ultimately helps athlete to work on it in next pratice session.

Importance of Limbering down:

1. It brings down to normal the body systems for example. It slowly controls the blood flow needed by the body as while doing exercises muscles were in demand of more blood supply and sudden stoppage of excessive supply of blood may cause pooling of blood, giddiness, sometimes collapse of nerves.

2. It helps in removing of the lactic acid from muscles which reduces the chances of soreness or stiffness. It reduces fatigue.

3. Stretching exercises relaxes the tired muscles.

4. Quickly stopping of activity may cause lead athlete to fever because of biological reasons (temperature of athletes body atmosphere varies). Therefore limbering down prevents athlete to fall in fever.

5. It improves or controls psychological aspects that are needed in normal social living.

6. In long run limbering down improves the performance of athlete as while limbering down athlete thinks of its mistakes done and mentally prepares and motivates himself to overcome those mistakes.

A warming up routine is particularly vital before any aerobic or anaerobic activity, because the heart, if launched into sudden action, reacts with abnormal rhythms, which can kill an untrained person. As you warm up, your body temperatures rises and the increasing need for oxygen in the newly exerting muscles stimulates a rise in the heart rate so that oxygenated blood can be pumped more quickly to the muscles. A arm-up makes exercise much easier. As blood surges into the ends of the muscles, forcing open new capillaries and raising body temperature, nerve endings are prepared for fast reaction, while the loosened joints & muscles expand their range of movement. E.g. stride length increases - a flexible body needs less energy to move. In short, warming up-exercises develop better blood circulation and also increase breathing rate of the participant. The muscles too get more flexible and efficient.

Meaning of warming up

- Warming -up is a small activity carried out in the preparation of the main activity.

- Warming -up exercises are those selected exercises which a player does before he takes part in the main activity.

- Warming-up is a period of preparing body, physically and mentally for a particular activity.

Thus a player who is thoroughly warmed up is not only able to put up a superior performance but can save himself from injuries too.

Duration: - The duration warming-up exercises should be according to age, sex, king of competition, its level, weather etc.

Types of warming up: -

Warming -up exercises are of two kinds: -

a) General warming -up b) Specific warming-up

a) General warming-up :- General warming -up meant for general physical preparation i.e. warming up the whole body, for the main activity.

General warming up consists of those exercises or movements that involve general body movement, jogging for sometime followed by loosening and stretching exercises, concluded with few sprints.

Aims:-

- Raise body temperature.
- Develop certain co-ordination.
- Readiness of physiological organs.
- Physical & mental readiness.
- It helps to acclimatize to environment.

b) Specific warming up:-

- Specific warming up is meant to prepare a body for a definite type of activity.
- It consists of exercises, which are undertaken after a general warming up, keeping in view the specific use of parts of body. These are done according to the game & the activity in view.
- It belongs to technical and tactical preparations.

Aims:-

- Get acquainted with the equipment used.
- Know the behavior of the balloon that surface.

- Gain confidence.
- Get toned up for the main task.
- Involvement of specific muscles.
- To avoid injury.

Specific warm-up for certain major games: -

Hockey: -

Hockey is a stick and ball game therefore all the motor movements are to be performed with stick either at a stationary position or moving with the ball in the hockey field.

The fundamental sills of the hockey are:-

1.dribble 2.push 3.hit 4.flick 5.scoop.

In order to perform the above written skills in an accurate war, a player needs a high level of neuron-muscular coordination, which can only be achieved by doing specific warming up exercises.

Few of which are written below: -

1. wrist rotation
2. dribbling
3. tapping
4. pushing
5. hitting
6. Scoops etc. All these can be done in specific warming -up to achieve optimum performance quickly

Football: - Now a day, football is also known as the game of uncontrolled passion. Every team want to be a winner and the team whose players have better skill, better coordinative ability, better tactics will be a sure winner.

The basic skills in the game of football are: -

I. Kicking

II. Dribbling

III. Heading

IV. Tackling etc.

Therefore the exercises performed in the specific warming up can be: -

1) Ball dribbling

2) Ball juggling

3) Kicking

4) Heading etc.

Basketball: - basketball is said to the world 's second fastest game, meaning every player has to physically fit, agile, technically &tactically sound. Thus specific warm up is important. The fundamental skills in the game of basketball are: -

1) Jump ball

2) Chest pass

3) Bounce pass

4) Low dribble

5) High dribble

6) Pivot foot

7) Jump shot

8) Lay-up shot

Exercises in the specific warming up can be: -

1) Shuttle running

2) Dribbling

3) Shooting or basketball practice. In basketball before any match is played all player are allotted time for practice on the ground.

4) Lay-up shoots

5) Dodging & fake practice etc.

6) Pivoting

Volley Ball:- Volley ball is a team game each team comprises of 6 players with 6 substitute players. These days volleyball has become fast and popular game.

The Fundamental skills in the game of volleyball are:-

(I) Service

(II) Smash

(III) Tip/Lift

(IV) Under arm lift

(V) Block

Specific warm up exercises include: -

(I) Service practice

(II) Smashing

(III) Lifting etc.

Judo: - Judo is a Japanese game, which means "the gentle way". A player of Judo is called 'Judoka' Judo involves has to hand or unarmed combat exercises that it concentrates mainly on throws allows-locks 7 strangles & requires a long 30 second fin.

The basic techniques used in Judo are: -

I) The throw

II) The Elbow lock

III) Griping

IV) Positioning

V) Pinning

VI) Choking

Specific Warming up: -

Before starting the main activity/competition the whole body has to be properly warmed-up in order to achieve optitum performance level quickly to avoid injury.

Specific exercises are: -

I) Proper strengthening of different muscles, i.e. muscles of upper and lower extremities both.

II) Throwing

III) Gripping

IV) Uchi Komi

Wrestling: - Wrestling is a barehanded comat sport in which two opponents try throw each other and pin their shoulders to the ground using holds & techniques. Wrestling is one of the oldest forms of combat sport.

The various skills used are: -

(I) Gut wrench

(II) Double leg tackle

(III) Hip toss

Specific warming up exercises can be: -

(I) Grounding practice

(II) Pivoting practice

(III) Pushing

(IV) Gripping

Athletics:-

Track and Field is primarily an individual sport, consisting approximately of 30 different events, which i.e. sprints, middle distance, long distance and obstacle races jumping and throwing. Therefore an athlete has to do specific warm up keeping in view the type of event in which he is to complete.

(I) Jogging

(II) Strides

(III) Sprinting

(IV) Stretching exercises of different body part. E.g.

(a) Leg Stretch

(b) Arm stretch

(c) Trunck stretch

(d) Ankle rotation

(e) Hip rotation

(f) Twisting

(g) Moving the hands forward & backward while standing.

5

Biomechanics of Muscles

It has been argued that the single most important topic in the field of exercise physiology is the muscular system. While it is indeed true that muscles will fail to function normally if innervation is withheld or if the circulation is impaired, the fact remains that the total organism is put into motion and remains there because of the action of skeletal muscles. In a very real sense, then, it is essential that the structure and function of muscles be understood in some detail, so that an adequate explanation may be available concerning practical matters of exercise and training. This chapter will deal with factors surrounding the structure and function of skeletal muscle.

STRUCTURE OF MUSCLE

The student of kinesiology will immediately recognize that human skeletal muscles are arranged in a variety of configurations, depending upon the function for which they are intended. It is common to think of muscle as being composed of fibres that seem to run directly from tendon to tendon, such as in the biceps brachii, but in reality a large number of muscles in the human body are small, with their fibres arranged in a variety of ways. In one example, the *longitudinal type,* the fibres run approximately parallel to the long axis of the muscle, although they may not reach the entire distance covered by the muscle. In the linguistics muscle, for instance, the fibres need not be very long, running from the spinous processes of vertebrae to the transverse process and lateral surfaces of the ribs, a distance of only a few inches.

In the *unipennate* form, the fibres approach the tendon from only one side, as occurs with the tibialis posterior muscle, whilc the *bipennate* muscle has fibres converging on both sides of the tendon, as illustrated by the rectus femoris muscle. An example of the *multipennate* muscle is shown by the deltoid, where internal collagenous sheets divide the muscle into three parts, thus providing a mixture of the first two pennate forms. The advantage gained by these variations is easily seen, as there is provided a means for initiating movement, particularly for joints that may be involved with large masses, such as the trunk where the surface area is large, or in other specialized areas of the body where range of motion may not be great. One can compare the function of the trapexius with that of the biceps to realize the great differences in joint function that are served. The fact that the fibres in penniform muscles shorten less than longitudinal muscles probably only attests to the types of functions they are intended to serve.

The contractile portion of the muscle gradually gives way to connective tissue, which is continuous with the tendons of origin and insertion, and forms a rigid adherence to bone so that it may bear the full tension of contraction. As the structure of the tendon interweaves with the muscle, the collagenous threads form a network that binds the muscle itself together without interfering either with contraction or the fibre arrangement. The individual fibres are surrounded by *endomysium,* and a group of as many as 150 individual fibres, called a *fasciculus,* is bound together by *perimysium.* The whole muscle is encased in a connective tissue sheath called the *epimysium.*

FIBRE CHARACTERISTICS

In order to understand the complexities of total muscle contraction, it is first necessary to understand the detailed characteristics of the muscle fibre. Since the thrust of exercise physiology necessarily implies external work and usually movement, the discussion will be restricted to skeletal muscle, rather than smooth muscle or cardiac muscle, although the latter will receive special attention in .

As noted in skeletal muscles are composed of rather large numbers of fibres, amounting in large muscles to many thousands. In fact, individual fibre count of an older adult engaged in a lifetime of hardwork revealed that the biceps contained over 316,000 fibres, arranged in more than 3,300 facicles. This would leave nearly 100 fibres to each fasciculus for that muscle. The fibres themselves range in size from 10 to 100 microns in diameter (.01 to .10 mm or 100,000 to 1, 000,000 A), and are surrounded by the *sarcolemma, the* muscle cell membrane found just beneath the endomysium.

It is not the individual fibre per se that is crucial to understanding of the contraction characteristics of muscle so much as it is the constituency of the fibre. The fibres have the striated appearance that characterizes skeletal muscle, and a single fibre is composed of a number of *myofibrils.* The myofibril can be further resolved into a series of repeating light and dark patterns known as *sarcomeres.* The sarcomere reveals that it consists of protein microfilaments, the thin filaments of *actin* and the thick filaments of *myosin.*

The sarcomere is further illustrated in an electron micrograph of the leg muscle of a frog. The persistent striations of the myofibrils result in a repeated pattern of light and dark areas. The less dense filaments of actin form a light zone, called the *I-band,* and the thicker filaments of myosin, which includes some overlapping by actin, from the more dense *A-band.* The actin filaments themselves arise from a membrane called the Z-line, which clearly marks the boundary between adjacent sarcomeres. The Z-membrane, in addition to actin, contains another protein, *tropomyosin, which* plays a significant role in the actual contraction sequence, as will be seen subsequently. Thus, the I-band is composed of actin and goes from Z-line to the beginning of the myosin filament, whereas the A-band consists of the myosin filament plus an overlapping portion of actin. The centre of the sarcomere contains a lighter zone, called the *H-zone,* the size of which depends upon muscle length, or the extent of overlap of thick and thin filaments. In the centre of the H-zone is a region of low density, the *pseudo H-zone,* and a dark centre portion called the *M-line.* It is possible that the M-line contains projections not made of myosin which are capable of lining together adjacent myosin filaments.

While it is attractive to present the structure of muscle almost in two-dimensional array, it should be stressed that muscle fibres, and therefore their myofibrils, are packed in rather high density as bundles, and hence should be thought of as three-dimensional. In fact, the thick and thin filaments are arranged in a six-sided (hexagonal) pattern, as shown in. In the region of overlap, which occurs in the A-band, the actin filament lies between three myosin filaments. Stated in another way, it can be seen that myosin lies symmetrically between six actin filaments. The question, then, centres around what characteristics actin and myosin have that permit the sarcomere to shorten during contraction.

Evidence is quite conclusive that projections, called *cross-bridges,* exist on myosin at regular intervals. Thus, at a given level on myosin, two of the cross-bridges project directly opposite each other. Rotating 60 degrees, the next set of projections occurs 143 A lower, continuing in this manner until finally the pattern repeats itself. This makes it possible for the myosin filament to interdigitate with the actin filament, which in turn is thought to have receptive "active sites". Actin, however, consists of beadlike molecules connected together in a double helical form, as shown in. Presumably, this arrangement would make it possible for actin to present the active sites to a variety of myosin filaments. The myosin molecule, on the other hand, consists of two parts, a head and a tail, as illustrated in. The tails, more appropriately termed *light meromyosin* (MM), become attached to each other to form a filament, and the heads, known as *heavy meromyosin* (HMM), project from the body of the filament. The HMM has the ability to interdigitate with actin, while LMM does not. Note that the heads on the two sides of the filament oppose each other, with a projection-free area in the centre; this corresponds to the pseudo H-zone, a region of especially low density. It will soon become clear that the placement of HMM in this manner makes it possible for effective shortening of the sarcomere to take place.

THE SLIDING-FILAMENT MODEL OF CONTRACTION

The most widely accepted model to explain the contraction of muscle is embodied into the sliding-filament concept. The major occurrence is for the Z-lines of the sarcomere to be drawn in toward the A-band, gradually narrowing and finally even eliminating the I-band, but without changing the length of the A-band. In this manner, the myosin filaments of the A-band retain a constant length, and the actin filaments are thought to slide over the myosin as the sarcomere approaches full shortening, perhaps even overlapping near the centre of the sarcomere, as shown in. Theoretically, this overlapping would place thc actin filaments on the one side in the way of effective movement on the other, and has been suggested as a possible explanation for the loss in tension experienced by muscles contracting in a shortened position. At any rate, the sliding is caused by a series of reactions between the HMM and the active sites on the actin filaments, so that the actin filament is pulled along, permitting the HMM to be released for reattachment at another site further along. It should be noted that the direction of pull is different on either side of the M-line, so that the movement of the actin filaments is always toward the centre in each sarcomere. Thus, the tension produced becomes proportional to the number of cross-bridges that can be formed between the A-and I-filaments. Acting in concert, the entire isometric tension of the muscle will be determined by the total number of interdigitating elements that are brought into play.

A MOLECULAR THEORY OF CONTRACTION

In order to bring the known elements of contraction together to form an integrated theory that not only explains the mechanical aspects of contraction but accounts for the energization process as well is a difficult task, since all aspects of the mechanism are not presently known. However, an important theory has been proposed which attempts to account for the movement of myosin heads as they move actin toward the centre of the A-band. This model, when modified slightly, helps us understand the contraction sequence.

The major premise upon which this theory rests is that an electrostatic bond is formed between the HMM of myosin and the actin filament, the latter of which contains, in addition to actin, *troponin and tropomyosin.*

In the presence of *calcium* (Ca^{++}), the HMM contracts, pulls the actin along one step, and then reextends for a second cycle. Schematically, this can be represented as in. Ionized *adenosine triphosphate* (ATP), a high-energy compound, is present at the end of the HMM, bearing a negative charge. At the base of the HMM is a fixed negative charge, which repels the negative charge on the ionized ATP. The enzyme ATPase which is capable of splitting ATP into *adenosine diphosphate* (ADP) and free phosphate (Pi) is also located at the base of the HMM, so that in the resting state this mobile HMM is extended, repelled by the similar charges. Bound ADP is present at an active site on actin and bears a negative charge. At rest, the complex of actin, troponin, and tropomyosin prevents interaction of the actin and mosin filaments, and relaxation is maintained.

The arrival of the nerve impulse causes the release of Ca^{++} from its bound state in the sarcoplasmic reticulum. This signals the release of free Ca^{++}, and by some reaction involving tropomyosin, troponin binds the Ca^{++} and removes the inhibition, permitting the liberated calcium ions to attach to the negative charge on the cross-bridge site of actin and the HMM. This forms an electrostatic depolarization and link formation, and the extended HMM contracts, moving the actin along towards the M-line. The sequences can be seen in.

The contraction of the mobile portion of the HMM brings the ionized ATP into the range of the ATPase, which breaks the ATP down into ADP and a phosphate ion, releasing energy. Thus, the energization sequence can be visualized in the following reaction:

ATP ADP + Pi+ free energy;

the bond is then broken between actin and myosin filaments. The ATP is quickly replenished by a fresh molecule of cytoplasmic ATP and the negative charge to the end of the HMM is restored. This results in electrostatic repulsion with the fixed negative charge and causes the HMM to be extended. As long as calcium ions are still present, the cycle will repeat itself, but during relaxation, when calcium is withdrawn into the sarcoplasmic reticulum, the HMM remains extended, and no electrostatic attraction occurs. In fact, special changes occur in the myofibrils themselves, which involve not only troponin and tropomyosin, but magnesium (Mg^{++}) and ATP as well MgATP). The role of magnesium seems to be that of binding ATP to myosin. The details of relaxation are not as clear as those of contraction, but the reader will find references in the literature to a *relaxing factor* system which account for the return of the sarcomere to resting length.

The amount of tension generated by each sarcomere is understandably small and will not be constant, because it will depend upon the amount of overlap of actin and myosin filaments. Increasing the number of myosin heads that can come into contact with actin will, up to a point, increase the amount of active tension that can be developed. The reactions described above occur at a rate of perhaps 100 cycles per second, so when it is realized that each myofibril contains a large number of sarcomeres, and each fibre contains a number of myofibrils, and, finally, the motor unit contains several muscle fibres, we see that, taken together, the maximum muscle tension must depend upon activating the largest number of sarcomeres through innervation of the greatest number of motor units. Whole muscle tension development will be described in the next chapter.

Nervous Regulation

The nervous control for activation of muscle has been discussed earlier, so it should be clear that normally functioning muscle must be supported by adequate nerve supply. Some of the consequences of inadequate or interrupted action potentials will be discussed later. It should be reiterated here that since the motor unit behaves on the basis of an *all-or-none law*, no direct procedure can be found for increasing sarcomere tension individually. Any increase in strength must therefore depend upon supplying nerve impulses of sufficient intensity to recruit the maximum number of motor units, and thus, the maximum number of muscle fibres.

Circulation

The great importance of the circulation to the effective functioning of the muscular system cannot be ignored, and a more complete treatment of peripheral circulation will be presented. This is not to suggest that the central circulation, represented by the cardiac output, is of any less importance. The point is that, for continuing functioning, the local muscles must receive appropriate oxygen supply and removal of waste products via blood flow through the muscle. Therefore, the extent of the capillary network is important to the development of muscular endurance. In addition, muscles contain *myoglobin,* a pigment that can combine with oxygen more readily, and at lower partial pressures, than blood. Myoglobin may act as a temporary oxygen store in muscle, available in small amounts during periods when normal flow may be interrupted. Some muscles contain more myoglobin than others, and therefore under histologic examination appear redder. It is felt that such muscles are better equipped for endurance activity than the paler muscles, whose function seems better suited for more rapid, hence anaerobic, action.

Fibre Types. The reader should be aware of terminology that is in use to designate various fibre types in human skeletal muscle. Rather than simply designating muscle fibres as red and white, it is preferable to refer to their *fast twitch* (FT) and *slow twitch* (ST) characteristics. While both types are mixed in human muscles, a predominance of one over the other may exist, which would impart a characteristic colour. More important, however, is the fact that the FT fibres (white) are more capable of high speed activity of short duration, while the ST fibres (red) seem better able to sustain more long term endurance activity. The reason for this difference is that the FT fibres have high myosin ATPase activity and high glycolytic capacity, while the ST fibres have low myosin ATPase activity and low glycolytic capacity. Translated into functional terms, this means that the ST fibres are best suited for long term endurance activity, and the FT fibres for high speed or sudden muscular contraction.

Energization

The matter of energy supply, a central issue in the study of exercise physiology. The primary energy source is various foodstuffs in the diet, and the energy released is converted to ATP. Thus, the ATP is an essential ingredient in the metabolism of cells and, of course, the contraction of sarcomeres. The release of energy and consequent production of ADP [equation (2-1)] stimulates the resynthesis of ATP. This is accomplished by *creatine phosphate* (CP), according to the following reaction:

$$ADP + CP = ATP + creatine.$$

Since a major source of energy is carbohydrates in the diet, the presence of *glycogen* in muscle is of major importance. It will be seen that glycogen granules are intimately associated with the myofibrils, hence are a primary source of energy. Since the major portion of ATP will eventually be extracted in the *mitochondria,* it is also interesting to note their ready supply in the cytoplasm of the cell supporting the myofibrils.

HEAT PRODUCTION IN MUSCLE

The contraction of muscle causes the production of heat to increase greatly beyond resting values. This increase of heat takes place in conjunction with the events that precede contraction, the rise in tension brought on during isometric contractions or the shortening phase of isotonic contractions, and finally the events associated with relaxation and recovery. Thus, there are four phascs of heat production in muscle.

1. *Actication heat.* Activation heat is the heat production attributed to the dissociation of calcium from its bound state in the sarcoplasmic reticulum. It follows depolarization and precedes actual tension development, which means that it begins during the latent period.

2. *Shortening heat.* The heat generated during the shortening or contraction phase of an isotonic contraction is identified with bond formation of the H-meromyosin and actin filaments. This will continue during the sliding of the actin along the myosin filaments as new links are formed. Shortening heat is independent of load but proportional to the distance of shortening. There may be additional *maintenance heat* produced during an isometric contraction, associated with ATP breakdown steadily, preventing the slipping of actin filaments.

3. *Relaxation heat.* In an isotonic contraction, relaxation heat occurs with lowering the load and lengthening of the muscle during the relaxation phase of an isotonic contraction. The need of the contractile filaments at this point is for a supply of ATP for the relaxing factor system. No heat of relaxation is found unless the muscle relaxes under load. Stated in another way, if the load cannot pull out the muscle after it has shortened, work done is not degraded into heat.

4. *Delayed heat.* The above phases of heat production correspond to Hill's description of initial heat, and as such are associated with the contractile events themselves. Following this, however, the muscle liberates *delayed or recovery* heat once the mechanical events have been completed. Under aerobic conditions-that is, when oxygen is available in sufficient amounts during contraction-the oxidative delayed heat is approximately equal to initial heat and represents the oxidative processes of recovery, the resynthesis of high-energy phosphate compounds, thus restoring energy given off during the performance of work.

Mechanical and Dynamic Properties of Muscle

A great deal is known about the various mechanical properties of muscle, as they have been favourite topics of physiologists for decades. Some of the characteristics to be described are so "classic" in nature that they have become suitable subjects for laboratory experiments in undergraduate physiology courses. These experiments are ordinarily conducted on isolated vertebrate muscle, such as that of the frog. Considerable progress has been made in learning about muscle tissue, but the crucial tests for human physiology will come when more complete information is available on muscle characteristics in vivo-that is, in the intact organism, not only with normal blood and nerve supply but with the muscle or group of muscles exerting tension through the usual muscle-tendon-joint complex. This chapter is devoted to such inquiry and will present a wide variety of topics, ending with a section on muscle training and hypertrophy.

LENGTH-TENSION CURVES

The amount of tension that a muscle can obtain depends upon its initial length. The maximum tension generated is not at resting length but when the muscle is slightly stretched beyond *equilibrium length.* A muscle that is foreshortened is at some disadvantage, as the amount of active tension produced becomes reduced. Even lengthening has its own built-in limitations, for excessive stretching can result in a decrement of active force. Considering the position of the actin just filaments, one can understand how extreme stretching can place actin just out of reach of the myosin cross-bridges. The shortened sarcomere is also at a disadvantage, as discussed. The lower curve in describes the tension produced when a resting muscle fibre is lengthened. The relationship between isometric tension and joint angle for the measurement of human elbow flexion is shown. Changing the joint angle effectively alters the muscle length, and for this particular test it reveals that 115 degrees is the most effective angle (most appropriate muscle length) for obtaining maximal tests of strength. Force drops off on either side of this value.

FORCE-VELOCITY CURVE

The muscle has been examined for speed of shortening after being loaded. The relationship is curvilinear and has been found to be mathematically predictable. It is observed that under essentially isometric conditions, where the velocity is zero, the force becomes maximal. It is difficult to load intact human muscles in quite the same way as the frog sartorius muscle, although the *force-time* curves of hand-gripping muscles have been examined when the muscles have adopted a preliminary tension varying from zero to 30 kg (66Ib). These curves are. There is a curvilinear (exponential) nature to these curves also, the best force being obtained when the performer begins with very little or no preliminary tension. If he adopts some force to begin with, the velocity of contraction noticeably slows, and there is likely to be some reduction in the amount of maximum tension achieved.

ELASTICITY

For muscle to exert tension it must activate its contractile components, as discussed. What may not be apparent is that the effective force generated is dampened by viscoelastic properties of the muscle and tendon. These elements must first be overcome during the uptake of force. The result of their activity is a reduction in the force measured externally, as compared with actual forces created by the contractile elements themselves.

These elastic components are arranged both in series and in parallel and represent the portions of the muscle that do not contract. These are shown, where their effects on tension can be seen.

The *series elastic component* is so named because the elastic elements occur directly in line with the contractile components; it is thought that these elastic elements are located in the tendons into which the muscle fibres are inserted, and are probably present at the Z-line region of the sarcomere. The *parallel elastic component* does not lie in series with the contractile mechanism, but in parallel, located specifically in the sarcolemma. The effect of this elasticity on effective tension. The contraction of the muscle imparts a given force, as illustrated in (b), but this can be increased if, at the time of stimulation, the muscle is first given a quick stretch so as to pull out the elastic elements. The increase in measured tension, (c), results from the elimination of the elastic elements. These elements smooth out changes in tension, lessening to some degree the sudden force invoked by the act of contraction.

REACTION LATENCY

A term often employed in physical education and athletics is *reaction latency,* or *reaction time.* The latent period is the time elapsing between the onset of the stimulus and the initiation of response by the contractile mechanism. It represents the duration of the nerve impulse. The reaction time, on the other hand, may include other factors that makes its duration somewhat longer than pure latency. The typical method of measuring reaction time is to present the subject with a stimulus, either auditory or visual, which starts a timer. As soon as the subject is able, the initiates some movement, which immediately stops the timer. The elapsed interval is reaction time (RT).

It the mass to be moved is large, the RT is longer than if the mass is small. Thus, finger RT is shorter than leg RT, because included in the measurement is time for the muscle contraction to move the mass of the limb involved. Since more motor units must be activated to move the heavier leg than the lighter finger, there will be a slight delay while this is being accomplished. This has led to use of the concept of premotor and motor reaction time, in which we separate RT into two components, employing an electromyograph to detect the instant that depolarization of the muscle cell membrane occurs. The *premotor time* is the time that elapses from the onset of the signal to initiation of the muscle action potential, and *motor time* is the time remaining for the actual response to be initiated.

It should also be pointed out that the onset of the signal is usually external, a sound or light stimulus, so some portion of the response time must be taken up with signal detection, to be followed by descending motor patterns to the appropriate body parts. Having the performer make a choice usually lengthens RT appreciably while he sorts out extraneous stimuli and decides upon the correct ones. Reaction time may be subject to some learning over a series of trials, the amount of this learning being greater if the individual must take a choice between alternatives in his response. The actual act of moving the body or its limbs is not a part of reaction time, since this is usually referred to as *movement time*. The time consumed by a ball carrier to the line of scrimmage is preceded by his reaction time; the time it takes for the action to be completed once it has been initiated is movement time. It may seem surprising, but a number of experiments indicate a low correlation between reaction time and movement time. In other words, an individual who has a fast reaction time does not necessarily have a fast movement time.

SUMMATION OF CONTRACTION

Strength of contraction can be increased in two different ways. Since the *motor unit* is the basic contractile entity, consisting of the motor nerve and all of the muscle fibres that it innervates, then it follows, first of all, that the force generated can be increased by bringing more motor units into play. However, a second factor involves the rate at which individual motor units are contracting. If a muscle stimulus is followed by a second one before the first is over, the total tension produced is increased. Thus, increasing the rate of firing up to 60 per second successively increases the maximum tension, and is an example of *wave summation.* This principle is presented. However, at a firing rate of approximately 60 per second, the successive contractions fuse together-a state of tetanus; further increases in rate lead only to slight increases in maximal tension. The individual motor units that become active contract rhythmically, but it turns out that they are out of phase with each other and so contract *asynchronously.* This serves a useful purpose by making the overall contraction appear to be smooth, even during weak contractions.

STAIRCASE PHENOMENON (TREPPE)

When a series of maximal stimuli are delivered to a muscle below a frequency that would cause tentanus, an increase in the tension during successive stimuli occurs, resulting eventually in a uniform tension. This is known as the *staircase phenomenon,* or treppe, from the German word for *staircase.* Undoubtedly, some sort of activation facilitation within the sarcomere allows the actin and myosin filaments to interdigitate more effectively.

SITE OF MUSCULAR FATIGUE

Repeated muscular exertion will soon lead to a fatigued state, greatly reducing the ability of the muscle to contract. There seem to be three potential sites where the focus of the fatigue process comes together: (1) the synapses of the central nervous system, (2) the neuromuscular junction, or (3) the muscle itself. It is difficult to imagine how the central nervous mechanisms could actually become fatigued during voluntary effort, although the following type of experiment would seem to indicate otherwise: voluntarily fatigue a muscle by a series of maximal contractions and then stimulate it directly by electrical means. It will be observed that the muscle seems to respond with renewed strength. Merton, however, indicated that perhaps in humans some fibres are not under control of voluntary effort, and demonstrated that a muscle does not contract by electrical stimulation after it has fatigued by voluntary effort. Employing the adductor policies muscle of the hand, he compared voluntary strength with maximal tetani and found them equal. As strength declined during the exercise bout, electrical stimulation of the motor nerve did not restore the tension, thus suggesting that the site of fatigue was peripheral-that is, in the muscle itself.

Further support was given this position by the finding that muscle action potentials evoked by nerve stimulation were not significantly reduced even in extreme fatigue, meaning that the wave of depolarisation was successfully crossing the neuromuscular junction. Moreover, recovery from fatigue did not take place if circulation to the muscle was occluded. Asmussen has stressed that local muscular fatigue involves the many chemical reactions, both aerobic and anerobic, that are responsible for delivering energy to the contractile mechanism of the myofibrils. The events associated with metabolism and energy transfer will be dealt with in.

FORM OF THE UPTAKE AND RELEASE OF FORCE

There have been very few efforts to study the characteristics of muscle contraction in the human with normal innervation and all other mechanical factors which produce maximal effort intact. The question involves how fast a maximal contraction can be made and what is the shape of the contraction curve. The contraction curve of the uptake of force of a single maximal contraction of the hand-gripping muscles. The force reaches half its maximum in approximately .08 sec, and three-fourths its maximum in .15 sec. By .4 sec the contraction is essentially complete. This compares with the mechanical responses of mammalian skeletal muscle fibre to a single maximal stimulus of .04 sec for the gastrocnemius and .1 sec for the soleus. Remember the earlier discussion of the slow twitch red and fast twitch white muscles reflecting different capacities, and the role of myoglobin in helping to make such a distinction. An interesting observation that can be made from that the greatest speed occurs in the early portion of the effort, but any increase in force later comes much more slowly. The release of tension, on the other hand, is much more rapid. Half the drop occurs in only .04 sec, and by approximately .15 sec resting tension has been achieved once again. Thus, release can take place some four times faster than contraction. As might be expected, the ability to exert force is affected by such things as prior activity and temperature. It is not surprising to find that immersion in cold water will reduce tension and markedly slow the rate of contraction, since this is a common experience encountered in cold weather. Its effect is to cut the speed of contraction approximately in half. A passive warm-up effect is less pronounced; that is, immersing the muscles in hot water does not lead to a very large change in contraction speed or strength. The release phase is lengthened by cold, but not by heat.

MUSCULAR FATIGUE

Since the turn of the century, there has been great interest in problems of muscular fatigue, and several experimental approaches have been tried. A complete understanding, however, has not been achieved. Such things as type of exercise and rate of work are crucial concepts. For example, is the exercise and rate of work crucial concepts. For example, is the exercise performed to be *isometric,* with no change in joint angle, or *isotonic,* employing a full range of motion? If the latter, is the resistance to be lifted a fixed amount, or some percentage of the person's maximum strength? Will he perform contractions according to some prescribed rhythm? If so, how much? If isometric, what is the criterion of fatigue? The topic is of practical significance to the teacher or coach, who should know something about the manner in which strength declines as a result of repeated effort.

The decline in strength is very rapid, dropping halfway from the initial value to a *steady state* or plateau in approximately 38 seconds. Contrast this curve with that for a series of maximal isotonic contractions, given at a rate of 30 per minute for six minutes. The drop-off to half strength under these conditions is 89 seconds; that is, fatigue is delayed at least three times longer employing rhythmic exercise (at the specified rate of contration) rather than nonrhythmic isometric exercise. Later on, the effect of isometric muscular contraction on the peripheral blood flow will be discussed but for the present it is clearly an advantage to have brief periods of rest, however small. Thus, the results of isotonic exercise are dependent upon the cadence used, so if the intercontraction rest interval is varied, the rate of fatigue and the level of steady state are both affected. This relationship can be seen. Reducing the rate of contraction from 30/min, as to 15/min raised the steady state appreciable from approximately 31 kg to 45 kg. On the other hand, increasing the cadence to 60/min reduced the fatigue level even more, down to approximately 20kg. Thus, as the intercontraction rest interval decreases, the steady state becomes lower, although the rate of this change is gradually becoming smaller. It is interesting to point out that so-called "complete fatigue" is absent when the subject is free to exert his maximum tension on each effort, rather than lifting a fixed weight.

In the latter case, it would eventually develop that the individual could no longer move the load. This is the common experience in weight-lifting exercises.

Physiologically, strength is related to the energy supplies available at the beginning of any exercise task. The muscles contain high energy reserves and will use them in proportion to the rate at which work is done, assuming-as we have in the present examples-that a constant cadence alternating between contraction and relaxation is employed. Thus, as the rate of exercise increases there will be a steadily diminishing ability of the muscles to be supplied with oxygen and to remove metabolic waste products. Apparently even a small rest between contractions permits some recuperation, for even with a cadence of 60/min a steady state is established well above zero. Initial occlusion of the blood flow (by a mechanical pressure cuff) is probably the only practical method of guaranteeing that complete fatigue will occur from isotonic exercise.

RECOVERY: THE STRENGTH DEBT OF EXERCISE

After about of exercise, the resulting decrement must be paid back in the recovery period. This is payment of the *strength debt*, analogous to the oxygen debt that involves the oxidative processes of recovery from exercise. The strength debt, or recovery, from fatiguing work has not received the same attention as the exercise phase itself, even though a number of practical problems in dealing with training and adjustment to optimal working conditions are involved. In a study by H.H. Clarke et al., subjects isotonically exercised the elbow flexor muscles until fatigue occurred when lifting a load equal to three-eighths of their strength. The recovery curve showed an initial rise during the first two minutes, followed by a slower gain for the next ten, so that recovery was still not complete for most subjects two hours after the cessation of exercise. Lind found fast and slow components in the ability of subjects to perform additional static contractions following fatigue.

The progress of recovery from isometric and istonic exercise is difficult to compare, since the two exercise forms can easily result in quite different levels of fatigue. However, this can be controlled, so that the pay off of the strength debt can begin at about the same value.

Recovery from exercise is quite rapid; in fact the gain in the first minute is appreciable, being 72 per cent for the isotonic conditions and 58 per cent for isometric. After this first minute the recovery from isometric is about 35 percent faster than from isotonic. This points out the finding-typical of experiments of this sort-that the recovery process consists of two components, one operating during the very early time period, the other controlling events later.

RESIDUAL MUSCULAR SORENESS

One of the handicaps associated with the resumption of exercise after an extended layoff is the usual experience of soreness in the exercised muscles. It ordinarily appears anywhere from 8 to 24 hours after activity and can be rather debilitating. This *residual muscular soreness* during exercise. Residual soreness may last for several days, depending upon the degree of exercise and the type of activity engaged in, and there is the assumption that no acute injury has occurred, since this would be reflected in immediate symptomatology.

The causative factors are not known, although minute tears in the muscle and connective tissue have been implicated, as well as an increase in extra or intercellular fluid, and the existence of tonic muscle spasms. Apparently not just any form of exercise leads to the same degree of residual soreness. Talag found the eccentric phase of exercise to produce the most pain.

6

Foundation of Sports Injuries

Design and Fabrication

(i) Principles used to design protective pads

(a) Mechanical structuring-forces are reduced through the use of a mechanical structure

(b) Channelling-forces are channelled away from anatomical structures

(c) Restriction—range of motion is to prevent forces that cause injury

(iv) Dispersion-forces are dispersed over a larger area

(ii) Sound bio-mechanical and anatomical principles should be well thought out before a fabricated pad is placed on an athlete

Head and Facial Area

Helmets

Types

(i) Single or double air bladder

(ii) Closed-cell padding with air bladder

Selection

(i) Helmets can :

(a) Prevent skull fracture and conclusions

(b) Protect facial bones, eyes, nose, mouth, and ears

(ii) Mandatory for football, ice hockey, mens' lacrosse, baseball, soft-ball, bicycling, amateur boxing, and white water sports

Fitting

(i) Hair should be the length that the athlete will wear it for the season. If a haircut is done during the season, the helmet should be re-checked for proper fit.

(ii) Circumference of skull should be measured above the ears

(a) Most football helmet manufacturers will supply tape measure at no cost

(b) Manufacturer's taped measures will have suggested helmet size on reverse of tape

(iii) Proper sized shell is selected and front and back sizes and jaw pads are adjusted for a proper fit

(iv) Athlete should then:

(a) Put on helmet by tilting it backward and rotating it to the front while pulling it into position

(b) Spread the earflaps by placing the thumbs or fingers directly in the ear holes

(v) Helmet should be snug and Dover base of skull but not impinge the cervical spine when the neck is extended

(vi) Four-point chin strap should be used and be of equal tension and length on both sides

(vii) Proper fit in other helmets is achieved when a snug-fitting helmet does not move in one direction when the head is turned in the other

(viii) Riddell and AHI provide free educational materials on the care and fitting of helmets

(ix) Crown adjustment

(a) Press straight down on top of helmet

(b) Helmet should be 1-to-2-finger widths above the eyebrows

(c) Helmet should not move over the eyes

(x) Side to side

(a) Grasp the face mask pulling left then right; the helmet should not slip

(b) Jaw pads should not have any gaps between them and the face

(c) Ask athlete to look straight ahead and "pull" the helmet should not slip

(xi) Up and down

(a) Athlete should scalp hands behind the helmet and press forward

(b) Athlete should "bull" the neck and tug up and down on the face mask; the helmet should not slip

(c) Fitter should not be ale to place a finger

(xii) Each helmet should have:

(a) Detailed records that identify purchase date, use, reconditioning history, and certifications seals

(b) NOCSAE seal of approval adhered to the posterior right side of the helmet

(c) Date and tracking number engraved on the inside

(xiii) Each athlete should:

(a) Sign and date a statement that confirms he or she read the seal and have been informed of the risks of injury by improperly using the helmet or face mask when striking an opponent

(b) Statements should be signed, dated, and kept as part of the athlete's medical files

(c) Be given instructions in the proper use, fit, and care of the helmet

(d) Participate in a pre-season in-service program on safety

(e) Should read the NOCSAE seal

Selection and Fitting

(i) Major testing agencies include:

(a) Canadian Standards Association

(b) National Operating Committee on Standards for Athletic Equipment

(c) Sports Equipment and Facilities Committee of the American Society for Testing Materials

(ii) Those responsible for purchasing, fitting, and maintaining equipment must know certification standards for protective gear

(iii) Rules regarding legal equipment are established by:

(a) National Federation of State High School Association for interscholastic competition

(b) National sports governing bodies for international competition

(c) National Collegiate Athletic Association for intercollegiate competition

(iv) Football, baseball, and lacrosse helmets must have the NOESEA seal of approval permanently stamped ono rear of helmet; ice hockey helmets must have the CSA seal of approval; other helmets must meet ASTM standards

(v) When fitting protective equipment consider:

(a) Mandatory rules so proper insurance coverage is not compromised

(b) Body size, age, strength, physical development, and skill level of athlete

(c) Sport and position

(vi) Regardless of playing position or level of competition, all equipment issued must pass inspection in a court of law

Maintenance

(i) Inspect and recondition the equipment by professional reconditioners after each season

(ii) Check equipment on a weekly basis, and if damaged, replace immediately

(iii) Establish a master plan for purchasing, replacing, reconditioning, maintaining and tracking the equipment's use and age

(iv) Reconditioning/warranty standards for football helmet:

(a) ABS plastic shell helmets have a 2-year warranty

(b) AHI helmets should not be used more than 6 years

(c) All helmets should be reconditioned every-2 years

(d) Polycarbonate alloy shell helmets have a 5 years warranty

(e) Riddell helmets should not be used more than 10 years

Mouthguards

Selection

(i) Are mandatory and should

(a) Provide support to toothless space so partial dentures can be removed when appropriate

(b) Protect lips, cheek tissues, and gums

(c) number and severity of jaw fractures

(d) incidence of contusions

(e) risk of broken and chipped teeth, root and bone fractures

(ii) Mouthguards should:

(a) Cover all upper teeth except the last two molars

(b) Not hamper breathing

(c) Be durable, resilient, tasteless, odourless, resistant to tear, easy to fabricate

(d) Be visible to officials

(e) Stay in place when mouth is opened

Types

(i) Boxer-type guards made moulded rubber

(ii) Custom-fitted

(iii) Mouth formed—boil and dip

Fitting

(i) Place mouth-guard over upper dental arch

(ii) Rinse guard in cold a water to harden material

(iii) Immerse guard in boiling water for 20 to 30 seconds

(iv) Shake off excess water, but do not rinse in cold water

(v) Close mouth, but do not bring teeth together or bite down on guard

(vi) Suck as hard as possible for 15 to 25 seconds to mould guard around teeth

(vii) Check guard for imperfections on the bottom, and if present, select new guard and repeat the process

Face Guards

Types

(i) Heavy-gauge, plastic coated steel rod

(ii) Clear plastic

Selection

(i) No face mask should have less than 2 bars

(ii) Face guards must meet NOCSAE standards for strength and deflection

(iii) Eye shields can be attached

(iv) Depends on position played and desired protection

(a) Quarterbacks, running backs, and wide receivers wear an intermediate style for an unobstructed view

(b) Lineman wear full cage with middle bar to prevent eye, nose, and facial injuries from opposing players' fingers

The Lower Body

Pelvis, Hip, and Thigh

Selection

(i) Depends on sport

(ii) Presence of pre-exiting injury

Types

(i) Girdle type pad is most effective for football, ice hockey, field hockey, and lacrosse goalkeepers

(ii) Thigh and hips pads

(a) Hard polythene covered with layers of Ensolite

(b) Neoprene

(c) Air management pads

(iii) Male genital region is best protected by a protective up in the athletic supporter

Fitting

(i) Girdle with pockets can hold hip, thigh, coccyx and genital pads in place

(ii) Thigh pads

(a) Should be centred over the quadriceps muscle group

(b) Asymmetrical thigh pads should have flared edge placed on lateral aspect of the thigh

(c) Should be placed 6 to 7 inches above the patella

Knee Braces

Selection

(i) Depends on:

(a) Physician recommendations

(b) Research and fit

(c) Proper diagnosis of condition

(ii) Functional knee braces provide stability for:

(a) Tedonitis

(b) Patellofemoral inflammations

(c) Ligament instability

(d) Bio-mechanical inefficiencies

(iii) Rehabilitation braces limit and protect knee ROM post-operative and non-post-operative

(iv) Prophylactic braces are worn to prevent or reduce incidence of knee injury

Type

(i) Functional

(ii) Prophylactic

(iii) Rehabilitative

Fitting

(i) Braces range from custom fitted braces to off-the-shelf models

(ii) Should be fitted according to manufacturer's

Lower Leg Protection

Selection

(i) Depends on:

(a) Proper diagnosis of condition

(b) Physician recommendations

(c) Research and fit

(ii) Heel cups are used to reduce shearing and shock in the calcaneal region

(iii) Footwear selection is based on:

(a) Position

(b) Sport

(c) Playing surface

(d) Weather conditions

(e) Postural or mechanical problems

(iv) Shin guards should have high density pad covered by a moulded hard shell

(v) Commercial ankle supports:

(a) Comfort and support, will determine personal preference

(b) Should be used when ROM must be limited

(vi) Inner-soles made of Poron

(a) Provide a porous structure to absorb and disperse shock

(b) Can be used for an arthritic or diabetic foot

(vii) Semirigid orthotics

(a) Often used for fallen arches, pronated feet, or medial tibial stress-syndrome

(b) Provides a more stable and durable support for intrinsic foot structures

(viii) Rigid orthotics more effectively correct bio-mechanical malignant

(ix) Anti-shock heel lifts

(a) Use dense silicone mixture to cushion heel impact

(b) Can correct some bio-mechanical alignment

(c) Can relive strain on the Achilles tendon

Types

(i) Shin guards

(a) Hard, deflective plastic outer player with an inner layer of thin foam

(b) Plastic stays sewn into a felt material

(c) Hard, deflective plastic outer layer with an inner layer of thin foam

(ii) Inner-soles

(iii) Semirigid orthotics

(iv) Rigid orthotics

(v) Anti-shock heel lifts and cups

(vi) Footwear

(vii) Commercial ankle supports

(a) Lace-up brace

(b) Semirigid arthrosis

(c) Air bladder brace

Fitting

(i) Shin guards should extend from the tibial tuberosity and cover malleoli

(ii) Ankle supports and other protective equipment should be flitted according to manufacturer's guidelines

(iii) Footwear

(a) Shop at stores that employ professional sales people that work with the sport

(b) Athletes with a history of back, knee, ankle, or foot injuries may opt for a shorter multi-cleated design for stability and torsion forces

(c) Fit shoes at the end of the day or after practice

(d) Wear socks that would normally be worn during competition

(e) Fit shoe to longest lose

(f) Fit shoe to widest part of foot, usually forefoot

The Neck and Upper Body

Shoulder Pads

Types

(i) Flat type:

(a) Used when a great deal of mobility is needed

(b) Is light and allows full ROM at glenohumeral Joint

(ii) Cantilevered:

(a) Is often worn by running backs, linebackers and defensive linemen

(b) is bulkier and has a device disperses impact forces over wider area of the body

Fitting

(i) Ice hockey and lacrosse pads:

(a) Pads are also sized for fit by measuring from AC joint to AC joint

(b) Pads must protect AC joint, clavicles, sternum, and shoulder cap

(ii) Sternum pads, rib protectors, and deltoid pads can supplement shoulder pads for extra protection

(iii) Football shoulder pads:

(a) Pads must be inspected weekly for cracks, loose or lose screws, or broke nor torn pads

(b) Measure across upper back from AC joint to AC joint

(c) Companies provide sizing charts to assist in selecting correct size for athlete

(d) Tip of the inside shoulder and should extend over lateral aspect of shoulder

(e) Pads should cover both scapulae, the sternum, clavicles, and extend 2 inches below nipple line

(f) Axillary and chest straps should be snug

(g) Neck opening should not impinge soft tissues of neck or slip when arms are abducted

Shoulder Harnesses

Selection

(i) Based on side specific

(ii) May be interchangeable on either shoulder

(a) Sully Brace can restrict excessive motion

(b) Prevents AC separations, and anterior or posterior dislocations

Types

(i) Several varieties available can restrict excessive abduction and external rotation

Neck rolls and Collars

Selection

(i) Depends on position played

(ii) May protect players with history of receptive burn or stingers

Types

(i) Wedge pad

(ii) External collar bolted to the pads

(iii) Round collar

(iv) Cowboy collar

Fitting

rolls and collars should never place the athletes neck in a flexed position

(a) Place cervical vertebrae in a fixed segmented column

(b) Risk of facial loading, which may result in catastrophic head or neck injury.

(ii) Fit to prevent hyperextension and lateral flexion of cervical vertebrae

Elbow, Forearm, Wrist, and Hand Protection

Selection

(i) Depends on condition and severity of injury

(ii) Material selection may be limited by sport governing bodies

Types

(i) Elbow braces

(a) Neoprene

(b) counter-force

(c) Hinge

(ii) Wrist and hand protection

(a) When immobilization is needed for fractures or sever sprains

(i) Silicone and fibreglass in preferred over heavier material

(ii) Can be worn during competition in must sports if padded properly

(b) Materials may include orthoplast, aquaplast, and plastazote

Environmental Considerations

Predisposing Factors to Heat Illness

(i) Children up to 12 years of age because they:

(a) Gain heat rapidly from the environment

(b) Lack judgement to understand impending symptoms of heat illness

(c) Sweat less efficiently

(d) Scclimate more slowly

(ii) Adults 55 or older because they:

(a) Have thirst mechanism when they become dehydrated

(b) Have less body water due to a lean body mass

(iii) Wheels chair athletes who do not like to drink fluids because of the inconvenience of urination

(iv) Diabetes that is uncontrolled

(v) Drugs: alcohol, amphetamines, cocaine, hallucinogens, laxatives, or narcotics

(vi) Poor acclimatization, poor physical condition, or

obesity

(vii) Athletes with excessive muscle mass

(viii) History of heat illness

(ix) Medications: anticholinergics, diuretics, antihistamines, anti–beta—blockers, laxatives

(x) Heart disease or hypertension

(xi) Eating disorders

(xii) Electrolyte loss or dehydrated

Preventative Measures

(i) Weight records

(ii) Change practice time to a cooler time of the day

(iii) Cooling spray aperitive/competition

(iv) Gradual acclimatization

(v) Frequent fluid replacement readings

(vi) Temperature/humidity readings

(vii) Identify individuals with predisposing factors

(viii) Modify uniforms by wearing shorts, cut-off jerseys, no helmets, etc.

Causes

(i) Inadequate replacement of fluids

(ii) Evaporation of perspiration is blocked due to

(a) High humidity

(b) Protective equipment

(iii) Life-threatening medial emergency

(iv) All mechanisms for body cooling fail during later

stages

Heat Stroke

Signs and Symptoms

(a) Gait is unsteady

(b) Disorientation and irritability

(c) Profuse seating

(ii) Late stages

(a) Pulse is rapid and strong

(b) Breathing is shallow

(c) Blood pressure

(d) Core temperature to 106°F

(e) Unconsciousness

(f) Seizes

(iii) As condition deteriorates

(a) Glassy stare, pupils dilated

(b) Skin becomes hot, dry, and red

(c) Sweating ceases

Organization Facilies

(i) Call EMS

(ii) Rapid cooling of the body

(a) Remote equipment and clothing

(b) Sponge the body with cold water or ice the major blood vessels in the axilla, groin, and neck

(c) Place athlete in a cold place

(d) Monitor vital signs until EMS arrives

(e) Use of fan, if available, or fan the athlete with a towel

(iii) Transport to a hospital as quickly as possible, continuing to cool the athlete during transport

Heat Exhaustion

Signs and Symptoms

(i) Skin calories ashen and gray

(ii) Skin is wet, col, and clammy

(iii) Core temperature; usually will not exceed 103°F

(iv) Pulse is rapid and weak

(v) Dizziness, lethargic, headache, fainting

(vi) Nausea

(vii) Uncoordinated gait

(viii) Blood pressure is low even in an upright position

(ix) Respiration is rapid and shallow

Organization Facilities

(i) If conscious, have athlete ingest cold clear fluids

(ii) Place athlete in a cool area

(iii) Remove all equipment and unnecessary clothing

(iv) Cool athlete by spongin or towelling him or her with cool water, particularly in the axilla, groin, and neck areas

(v) Take core temperature every 8 to 10 minutes making sure it does not exceed 106°F

(vi) Call emergency medical service

(vii) Monitor vital signs until EMS arrives

Heat Cramps

(i) Caused by imbalance between water and electrolytes in body from perspiration

Signs and Symptoms

(i) Involuntary muscle spasms

(ii) Fatigue

(iii) Nausea, vomiting

(iv) Headache

(v) Body Skin remains moist and cool

(vi) Pulse and respiration are normal or slightly elevated

(vii) Skin remains moist and cool

Organization Facilities

(i) Rehydrate by drinking cool water

(ii) Ice the muscle on stretch

(iii) Athlete will generally not be able to return to participation that day

High-Altitude Pulmonary Edema

Cause

(i) Caused by lungs accumulating a small amount of fluids within the alveolar walls, which lead to pulmonary edema

Predisposing Factors

(i) Athlete of not acclimated to altitude

(ii) Athletes who are not native to or reside in the area

Signs and Symptoms

(i) Develops after symptoms of acute mountain sickness subside

(ii) Unconsciousness may occur·

(iii) Fatigue and muscle weakness

(iv) Shortness of breath

(v) Headache and chest pain

(vi) respiration

(vii) Irritating cough with bloody, forth spectrum

(viii) Fatigue and muscle weakness

Organization Facilities

(i) Give oxygen, if available

(ii) Return to lower altitude immediately

(iii) Condition resolves quickly at lower altitude

Frostnip

(i) Often identified first by those around you

(ii) Affects the tips of ears, nose, cheeks, chin, fingers and toes

Signs and symptoms

(i) Slow, painless onset

(ii) No permanent tissue damage

(iii) Sudden blanching or whiteness of the skin

(iv) Slow, painless onset

(v) As warmth and colour returns, tingling may occur

(vi) Skin may turn red as warming occurs

(vii) Areas affected may peel or blister within 24 hours

Organization Facilities

(i) Apply firm steady pressure with a warm hand

(ii) Blow warm breath on the area

(iii) Do not rub the Area

(iv) Hold the nipped fingertips motionless in the axilla

Deep Frostbite

(i) A medical emergency

(ii) Usually affects hands feet but can affect ears, nose, cheeks, and chin

Organization Facilities

(i) Skin may permanently remain red, tender, and sensitive to re-exposure to cold

(ii) Transport athlete to the hospital/medical ability develop within 2 to 3 weeks

(iii) Take person indoors and do RAPID re-warning

(iv) Remove all jewellery and rings from fingers

(v) Immerse body part in warm water in a but large enough so the body part does not touch the sides or bottom

(vi) Pain and burning sensation may last for several weeks

(vii) If conscious, have athlete drinks hot clear fluids

(viii) Dry area after thawing, cover each digit individually with sterile gauze, and then over the entire area with towels or a blanket

(ix) In severe cases blisters will form and gangrene may develop within 2 to 3 weeks

Signs and Symptoms

(i) Skin appears cold, solid, and numb

(ii) As re-warming occurs:

(a) Extremely painful after thawing

(b) Swelling caused by capillary damage and plasma leaking into the tissue

(c) Skin will turn purplish blue

(iii) Firm, hard mass upon palpation with underlying tissues being rigid

Superficial Frostbite

(i) Affects the skin and underlying superficial tissue of the ears, nose, cheeks, chin, fingertips, and toes

(ii) Often identified first by individuals around you

Treatment

(i) A medical emergency

(ii) Usually affects hands and feet but can affect ears, nose, cheeks, and chin

Signs and Symptoms

(i) Skin appears pale, hard, cold, and waxy

(ii) Firmness upon palpation with underlying deeper tissues soft and resilient

(iii) As re-warming occurs:

(a) Swelling caused by capillary damage and plasma leaking into the tissues

(b) Skin may permanently remain red and sensitive to re-exposure to cold

(c) Athlete will first feel numbness, then stinging and

burning sensations

(d) Skin will turn mottled blue or purple

(e) blisters may form

Predisposing Factors to Cold Injuries

(i) Fatigue or weakness

(ii) Inadequate protection from the cold or wind

(iii) Use of alcohol and other substances

(iv) Persons with Raynaud's phenomenon

(v) Inadequate diet and fluid intake

(vi) Restricted circulation from arterial disease or tight clothing, especially foot wear

(vii) Children:

(a) With asthma are prone to bronchoconstriction when breathing cold air

(b) Lose body heat faster than adults

(c) Are more prone to frostbite because of their enhanced peripheral vasoconstriction

(viii) Older adults are less able to adapt to cold from:

(a) Ability to vasconstrict peripheral arterials

(b) Rise in heat production during cold stress

Preventative

(i) Gradual acclimatisation

(ii) Replace fluids to avoid dehydration

(iii) Longer warm-up period during cold weather, or warm-up indoors when possible

(iv) Protect the body from heat loss within:

(a) Outer jacket

(b) Face mask and neck warmer

(c) Cap or hat

(d) Gloves

Causes

(i) Prolonged exposure to wet-cold conditions

(ii) Shivering through involuntary muscle contractions to generate heat ceases

(iii) Body heat loss exceeds body heat production

(iv) Vasoconstriction surface blood vessels prevent blood rom shunting to the skin

(v) heart, liver, brain, and endocrine organs

Altitude-Related Conditions Acute Mountain Sickness

Causes

(i) Caused by hypoxia at altitudes of 7000 to 8000 feet

Predisposing Factors

(i) Diet low in carbohydrates and high in sodium

(ii) Athletes who are not native to or reside in the area

(iii) Athlete not acclimated to altitude

Organization Facilities

(i) Return to lower altitude immediately

(ii) Give oxygen, if available

(iii) Condition resolves quickly at lower altitude

Signs and Symptoms

(i) Headache and dizziness

(ii) Insomnia

(iii) Nausea, vomiting

(iv) Fatigue

(v) Appetite suppressed

(vi) Tachycardia on exercises

(vii) Dyspnoea

Emergency Care

Unconscious Athlete

Causes

(i) Concussion

(ii) Respiratory distress

(iii) Metabolic disturbance

(iv) Syncope

(v) Drug overdose

(vi) Liver/kidney failure

(vii) Haemorrhage/shock

(viii) Cerebrovascular of cardiovascular malfunctions

(ix) Poising

(x) Seizure/epilepsy

(xi) Edema/infection affecting the brain-stem

Organization Facilities

(i) Determine level of consciousness through verbal and sensory stimuli

(a) Call the person's name

(b) Pinch soft tissue

(c) Tap your knuckles on his her sternum

(ii) Unless there are special circumstances, such as respiratory distress coupled with an inability to access the airway, the helmet should never be removed on the field when there is a potential head/neck injury

(iii) If individual does not respond

(a) Activate appropriate emergency medical system

(b) Immediately assess airway and circulation

(iv) Assume the presence of associate cervical spine trauma

(v) If airway is compromised and/or circulation is absent, stabilize the head and cervical spine and perform a log roll to position the athlete supine

(vi) Remove face mask if present. Note: if proper tools are not available CPR pocket mask can fit under face mask without having to remove it

(vii) If airway is intact and circulation is present, protect the athlete from further injury, perform a secondary survey, continue to monitor vital signs until emergency transport personnel arrive

CPR Emergencies

Causes

(i) Direct trauma

(ii) Electrical shock

(iii) Strenuous activity

(iv) Excessive alcohol or substance abuse

(v) Drowning

(vi) Suffocation

(vii) Heart anomalies

Organization

(i) Summon EMS

(ii) Follow standard first aid procedures for CPR

Signs and Symptoms

(i) Pain originating behind the strum, which may radiate into one or both arms, the neck, jaw, teeth, upper back, or mid-abdomen

(ii) Feeling of impending doom

(iii) Nausea

(iv) Shortness of breath

Obstructed Airway

causes

(i) Solid foreign object

(ii) Swelling in the throat

(iii) Back of the tongue because of unconsciousness

(iv) Fluid

Organization Facilities

(i) Total airway obstruction

(a) Summon EMS

(b) Follow standard first aid procedures

(ii) Partial airway obstruction

(a) Reassure the individual you are there to help

(b) Allow individual to cough up object

Signs and Symptoms

(i) Partial airway obstruction

(a) Allows for some air exchange

(b) Individual exhibits choking behaviours

(ii) Complete airway obstruction

(a) Allows no air to pass

(b) Individual is unable to cough, speak, or breath

External Haemorrhage

Causes

(i) Requires removal from participation and prompt management to avoid infection and risk of disease transmission

(i) Shearing force coupled with tensile or compressive forces leading to exposed skin would

Organization Facilities

(i) Apply direct pressure with sterile gauze compressing the tissue firmly

(ii) Elevate the injured area about the heart

(iii) Put on latex gloves before you attempt to control haemorrhage

(iv) Apply indirect digital pressure to slow arterial bleeding

(v) Remove gloves, carefully turning them inside out to avoid contact with outer surface

(vi) Discard all blood-soaked gauze and gloves in a properly labelled biohazard container

Internal Haemorrhage

Causes

(i) Results from direct or indirect trauma

(ii) May occur in the presence of disease states leading to organ rupture

Organization Facilities

(i) Maintain an open airway

(ii) Continue to monitor vital signs until the ambulance arrives

(iii) Activate EMS

(iv) Monitor vital signs

(v) Check for fractures, splint if appropriate

(vi) Treat for shock

(vii) Loosen any restrictive equipment or padding at the neck and waist

(viii) Anticipate vomiting; place the individual on his or her side with the head downward, provided a spinal injury has been ruled out

(ix) Keep the individual calm and quiet

Signs and Symptoms

(i) Low blood pressure

(ii) Rapid, weak pulse

(iii) Bleeding from the mouth, rectum, or other body openings, bloody fluid from the nose or ears

(iv) Blood in the urine or urine output

(v) Nausea and vomiting blood

(vi) Severe respiratory distress; rapid breathing, possibly shallow

(vii) Pale, cold and clammy skin with profuse sweating

(viii) Feeling of impending doom, restlessness, or anxiety

(ix) Dull eyes, dilated pupils that are slow to respond to light

(x) pain, tenderness, swelling, or discoloration at the injury site

Shock

Cause

(i) The inability of the heat to exert adequate pressure to circulate enough oxygenated blood to vital organs

(ii) Occurs as a result of:

(a) Vessel dilation leading to blood pooling away from vital areas

(b) Damaged heart

(c) Low blood volume from blood or dehydration

Predisposing Conditions

(i) Severe pain

(ii) Bleeding

(iii) Spinal injuries

Organization Facilities

(i) If you do not suspect a head or neck injury, or leg fracture, elevate the feet and legs 8 to 12 inches

(ii) If there are breathing difficulties, the individual may be more comfortable in a semi-recline position

(iii) With a head injury, elevate the head and

shoulders to reduce pressure ono the brain

(iv) In a suspected neck and/or spine injury keep the individual lying flat

(v) If the individual vomits or is unconscious, place the athlete on his or her side to avoid blocking the airway with any fluids. This allows the fluids to drain from the mouth

(vi) Do no give the athlete anything by mouth

(vii) Monitor vital signs every 2 to 5 minutes until the ambulance arrives

(viii) Active EMs immediately

(a) Control any major bleeding and monitor vital signs

(b) Secure and maintain an open airway

(ix) Splint any fractures to reduce pain and limit shock

(a) Raise the leg only after it has been properly immobilized

(b) With a leg fracture, keep the leg level while splinting

(x) Move the individual to a warm environment

(a) Maintain body heat

(b) Remove any wet clothing if possible, and cover the individual with a blanket

Fractures and Dislocations

Causes

(i) Axial compression

(ii) Tensile forces that may or may not be combined; with shearing forces

Organization Facilities

Principles of Splinting

(i) Establish an open airway and complete the primary survey

(ii) Check the distal pulse and sensation

(a) if pulse is weak, check for internal haemorrhage

(b) If sensation is altered, summon EMS

(iii) Remove any clothing and jewellery around the injury site. Clothing should be cut away with scissors to avoid moving the injured area

(iv) Cover all wounds, including open fractures with sterile dressings and secure them

(v) Do not attempt to push the bone ends back underneath the skin

(vi) Pad the splint to prevent local pressure

(vii) Apply minimal in line traction and maintain it until splint is in place and secured

(viii) Air splints should not be used for an open fracture

(ix) Splint firmly, but do not impair circulation

(a) Re-check distal pulse and sensation after applying splint

(b) Check vital signs

(c) Arrange transport to a medical facility

(x) Immobilize the joint above and below the fracture site

(a) With such injuries, immobilize in the position you

find the limb in, moving it as little as possible during splint application

(b) If pain with gentle traction or the limb resists positioning, splint in the position found

(c) Severely angulate fractures should not be straightened unless it is absolutely necessary to incorporate limb into splint

Types of Splints

(i) Rigid splints are commercially available and are:

(a) Made of wood, aluminium, wire, cardboard, or plastic

(b) Designed in specific shapes for upper and lower extremities

(ii) Choice of splint is determined by site of fracture and availability of splinting materials

(iii) Pneumatic splints are soft and pliable prior to inflation and:

(a) Become rigid once inflated

(b) Can have a radiograph through it

(iv) Vacuum splints

(a) Work by removing air from the splint, causing a rigid supportive structure

(b) Can have a radiograph though it

(v) Traction splints

(a) Provide counter pull to immobilize bone ends and prevent further injury

(b) Immobilize long bones

(vi) Improvised splints

(a) Be light yet rigid

(b) Can be made from a cardboard box, magazine, newspaper, or shin guard

(c) The surface next to the skin should be padded

(d) Should and below the injury

Epiphyseal Fractures

(i) Account for over 15% of all fractures to adolescents

(ii) Classified in Salter–Harris categories according to risk of disruption of blood supply and growth arrest

(a) Type I: complete separation of epiphysis, no fracture through bone

(b) Most II: most common, involves the plate and a triangular segment of the metaphysis

(c) Type III: plate injury extends through articular cartilage into the joint

(d) Type IV: fracture extends through articular cartilage into the joint, and into the metaphysis

(e) Type V: crushing injury to epiphyseal plate

Organization Facilities

(i) Type I and II: managed with immobilization and have a good prognosis if the blood supply is intact

(ii) Type III and IV: managed with immobilization and internal fixation, however, prognosis for Type IV is poor

(iii) V is managed with non—weight-bearing g for 3+ weeks to prevent compression also and has a poor prognosis

Spinal Cord/Neurologic Injuries

Causes

(i) May result in life-threatening and/or catastrophic injuries to the spine central nervous system

(ii) May occur secondary to head trauma

Signs and Symptoms

(i) Pain on palpation

(ii) Burning pain that radiates

(iii) Weakness in a myotome

(iv) Reduced or absent reflexes

(v) Complete paralysis

(vi) Numbness, tingling, or loss of sensation in a dermatome

(vii) Muscles spasm

Management

(i) Observe body position

(ii) Assess level of consciousness

(iii) Determine presence of head, neck, or back pain

(iv) Assured pupil size, reactivity, and movement

(v) Check eyes, nose, and ears for the presence of blood and/or fluid

(vi) Palate spine and skull

(vii) Functional assessment: memory, cognitive function, behaviour, balance, and coordination

(viii) Assess neurologic function: cranial nerves and spinal nerves

(ix) Unless there are special circumstances, such as respiratory distress coupled with an inability to access the airway, a helmet should never be removed on the field where there is a potential head/neck injury

(x) Immobilize on spine board with constant stabilization of the head, neck, and spine

(xi) When vital signs are compromised CPR must be initiated immediately after positioning the athlete on the spine board

(a) Many CPR pocket mask airways can be slipped under the face mask without having to remove it

(b) Special sport specific equipment may have to be removed to perform ventilation, but should not be removed before spine-boarding the athlete

7

Mechanics of Musculo-Skeletal Injury

It is usually observed that all injury leaves pain in the memory and for Olympic-calibre athletes, the memory often is not limited to the injury itself, but frequently includes the lifelong pain of lost opportunity. Injury can affect peak performance - through the loss of a millimetre or fraction of a second- and be the deciding factor in being chosen for an Olympic medal. As tragic as injury can be in denying an athlete the joy of Olympic competition, so too is Olympic history replete with stories of courageous athletes who have overcome injury to achieve the enduring glory of Olympic success.

Al Oerter, in Tokyo in 1964 won the third of his four gold medals by ignoring the pain of a dislocated cervical vertebra and torn rib cartilage and hurling the discus an Olympic record distance of 60.54m. In receiving his unprecedented third gold medal, Oerter said, these are the Olympics. You die for them.

Injury is an undeniable facet of athletic life. Individuals across the spectrum of competitive levels, from recreational athletes to Olympic competitors, are subject to the limitations and disappointments imposed by musculoskeletal injury. Elite athletes, however, are particularly susceptible to the physical, emotional and economic costs that injury exacts. Though these costs are in consequential for minor injuries, they can be overwhelming in cases of devastating injury that make it impossible, either temporarily or permanently, for an athlete to train and compete.

Lessening the chance of injury and facilitating the treatment and recovery of injured athletes requires and interdisciplinary approach that includes consideration of the anatomical, physiological, medical, kinesiological, psychological and mechanical aspects of athletes and their competitive environments. The injury-related problems of elite athletes are not addressed optimally by each discipline acting in isolation. The interdisciplinary team may include medical professional, physical therapists, athletic trainers, sport scientists, psychologists, coaches and athletes.

Each of these professionals brings a specific perspective to the challenges of dealing with injuries to athletes. In addition to these individual perspectives, musculoskeletal injury can be viewed from many different general perspectives, including historical, epidemiological, economic, psychological and biomechanical.

EPIDEMIOLOGICAL PERSPECTIVE

Epidemiology- the study of the incidence, distribution and control of disease and injury- documents the frequency and distribution of a particular injury in a given population. With the large number of participating nations, the huge array of sporting events and numbers of participating athletes, and the scatter in data-collection procedures, comprehensive injury data for Olympic athletes do not exist. While isolated reports of injuries to specific groups of Olympic competitors are available comprehensive documentation of injuries to Olympic athletes is unavailable and may remain so in light of the logistical constrained to gathering such data. In the general population, many injuries are never officially recorded. Thus published injury statistics are underestimates of the true injury toll. This is undoubtedly true for Olympic athletes as well; it is highly likely that many more injuries happen than are officially recorded and reported.

Historical Perspective

Archaeological evidence suggests that musculoskeletal injury is as old as itself. As well, injury is endemic to athletic lore, as illustrated in the legendary tale of Phidippides, who fell dead on the plain of Marathon after running 40 km and proclaiming the news of the Atheneum victory over the Persian forces of Dariuys the Great.

Injuries always have been and will continue to be a part of the athletic experience for participants at all level of sport. Despite the inevitability of injury, athletes have benefited greatly from medical progress in the 20th century. Advances such as clinical arthroscopy, pioneered by Bircher in the early 1900s, presaged an age in which rapidly developing technologies would render tractable many problems that were previously impossible to solve. Not long ago, laser surgery, advanced imaging techniques, micro- surgery and computer- or robot-assisted surgery were dismissed as futuristic dreams. Such medical advance, combined with remarkably improved rehabilitative programs, not provide new hope where previously there was only despair. Many athletes, who in earlier times would have been unable to compete due to injury, are now able to fulfil their dreams of Olympic participation.

Economic Perspective

While injury exacts physical and emotional coasts,

the economic consequences of injury are often overlooked. Such costs include direct costs and morality costs. Since death due to athletic injuries is rare, the last of these costs is of minor consequence. The combination of direct and morbidity costs resulting from athletic injuries, however, is considerable. For an event such as the Olympic Games, these costs can account for a significant portion of the event's budget. At an individual level, the costs can be even more catastrophic, especially in cases where one's economic livelihood is predicated on his or her athletic success.

Psychological Perspective

The most noticeable consequence of injury is the direct, physical damage to the body's tissues. Less obvious, and arguably no less important, are the psychological consequences that accompany musculoskeletal injury. Injury-related psychological factors can be involved before, during and after the actual injury, and can influence the likelihood and severity of injury, and the course of treatment and rehabilitation.

The psychological profiles of highly competitive, Olympic-calibre athletes differ in many ways from those of the general population. Psychological attributes such as high motivation, pain tolerance, goal orientation and exemplar physical training habits can benefit one's performance. On the negative side, elite athletes may be predisposed to a higher sense of loss, greater threat to their self-image, and harbour unrealistic expectations and a desire for a quick recovery from injury. While some psychological factors are common to athletes across a wide range of athletic events, the risk of injury also is clearly event-dependent. An Olympic alone skier or boxer, is much likely to suffer an injury than a participant in events such as curling of archery. Psychological factors affecting athletic performance and injury should be neither underestimated nor ignored.

Biomechanical Concepts

Movement is inherent to life and the quintessential element of our being. Without movement there would be no life. Some forms of movement developed to ensure survival, and others evolved as a means of expression. Athletic movements, in particular, are among the most demanding of all those imposed on the human body's framework.

Assessment of movement from a descriptive perspective falls within the area of mechanics known as kinematics. Kinematic analysis of movement involves five -primary descriptive variables.

1. acceleration indicating how quickly the velocity has changed.

2. velocity measuring how fast something has moved.

3. displacement describing what movement has occurred;

4. position or location.

5. time temporal characteristics of movement.

Movement description provides a useful tool for coaches and athletes in assessing the movement demands of their respective sports. Description alone, however, has limitations, and a comprehensive analysis of a movement pattern or skill also requires knowledge of the forces that produce the movement. Analysis of the force-related characteristics of movement falls within the area of mechanics known as kinetics.

Biomechanical perspective

Off all scientific disciplines, physics and its subdiscipline, mechanics, are arguably most central to the study of injury, since most injuries have mechanically related causes. Forces and force-related factors are the prime agents that determine the likelihood and severity of injury. The nature of an injury and its treatment rests on the effective integration of biological and mechanical knowledge. Interdisciplinary biomechanics is ideally positioned to provide this integrated perspective. In the case of musculoskeletal injury to prevention, diagnosis and severity. The goal is to mitigate the negative effects of injury and allow athletes at all levels to maximize their performance potential.

Force and Pressures

Body movements are produced and controlled by forces acting both within the body and upon body from external sources. These forces, in addition to modulating movement patterns, also act on tissues in the body. Under most conditions, these forces are well tolerated by the body's tissues in the body. Under most conditions, these forces are well tolerated by the body's tissues. Indeed, force is central to optimal growth and development of tissues, especially those such as bone that provide structural support. But when forces exceed a tissue's ability to withstand the load, injury occurs. Force therefore is the most fundamental element in injuries.

Force is defined as the mechanical action or effect applied to a body that tends to produce acceleration. The standard unit of force is the newton, which is defined as the amount of force necessary to accelerate a 1 kg mass at 1 m. Forces pertinent to injury analysis include those that act in or upon the human body, and include gravity, impact, musculotendinous forces, ligamentous forces that stabilise joints, and forces applied to bones. For all injury related forces, seven factors combine to determine the nature and severity of the injury. These factors are:

1. rate how quickly is the forced applied?

2. variability is the magnitude of the force constant or variable over the application interval?

3. duration over what time interval is the force applied?

4. direction where is the force directed?

5. location where on the body or structure is the force applied?

6. magnitude how much force is applied?

Injury often occurs when one object impacts with another, such as when an ice- hockey player collides with an opponent or with the boards. Impact also occurs when an object such as a ball contacts an athlete. A sharp object contacting the skin with a given force level will cause a different injury than a blunt object that impacts the skin with a similar force. In general, as the area of force application increases, the likelihood of injury decreases. This relation between force and application area is measured by pressure, which is defined as the applied force divided by the area over which the force is applied. The standard unit of pressure is the pascal, defined as 1 N force applied to an area of m^2 . In cases where forces are applied to structures over a relatively small area, a more convenient unit of pressure is the megapascal, equal to a 1N force applied to 1 mm^2.

Viscoelasticity

A material is said to be elastic if it has the ability to return to its original shape when a mechanical load is removed. Bone, is elastic since the slight bending induced by a compressive load disappears when the load is removed and the bone returns to its original shape. Body tissues are elastic within their physiological ranges of normal movements, but tissues that are deformed beyond the elastic limit are injured.

The mechanical response of any material depends on its constituent matter, Biological tissues generally have a fluid component and therefore are influenced by the principle of fluid mechanics. One of the most important of these principles posits that the response of a tissue depends, in part, on the rate at which the tissue is deformed. The tissue is described as being strain-rate dependent. A tendon, that is stretched quickly will respond differently than the same tendon stretched more slowly. Specifically, the quickly stretched tendon will be suffer, stronger and will absorb more energy if taken to its point of rupture.

Tissues possessing these conjoint properties of elasticity and viscous strain-rate dependency are called viscoelastic tissues. The nature of a tissue's viscoelastic response plays an important role in the path-mechanics of injury.

Stress, Strain and Stiffness

When examining human movement, envisioning the body's segments as rigid links is sometimes useful. Such rigid-body formulations make assumptions of non-deformability, fixed centre of mass, and material homogeneity. Although biological materials are deformable the limitations imposed by the simplifying assumptions of a rigid-body model are generally acceptable for quantifying movement mechanics. In exploring the biomechanics of musculo-skeletal injury, however, tissues must be considered as deformable solids since most injuries involve some amount of material deformation. In viewing bodily tissues as deformable solids, it is essential to understand the concepts of mechanical stress and strain.

A tissues loaded by an external force develops an internal resistance. The amount of resistance depends on the material properties of the tissue. In the case of skin, the resistance may be quite low. Bone, in contrast, will develop considerable resistance. This internal resistance is mechanical stress and is calculated by, where F is the magnitude of the load, and A is the tissue cross-sectional area over which the load is distributed. Stresses are classified as one of three types: tension, compression or shear.

Tension stress develops in response to tensile loads that seek to elongate, or stretch the tissue. Compression stress results when the load pushes the ends of the tissue together. Shear stress occurs when parallel forces act to produce an angulation or slippage between two surface.

Tissue typically change their shape in response to loading. This change is called a deformation and is measured as a mechanical strain. Just as there are three principal stresses, the deformational response for each stress produces a corresponding principle strain. Tensile strain is a stretching or elongation of the tissue. Compressive strain produces a decrease in the longitudinal dimensions of a tissue, such as when a vertebra is subjected to a compressive load.

Biological tissues have complex relations between stress and strain. Skin deforms readily under relatively low forces, whereas bone develops considerable internal resistance and deforms little. The responses of connective tissues such as tendon, ligament and cartilage fall between these two extremes. The relation between stress and strain can be visualized by plotting stress as a function of strain. The ratio provides a single numerical value describing the relation between stress and strain. This ratio it termed the stiffness of the material. Bone is relatively stiff and deforms little as loads are applied; by comparison, tendon is less stiff than bone. Typically, the mechanical responses of biological tissues are not linear throughout their physiological ranges, as explained in the next section.

Modes of Loading

During athletic activities, body tissues are continuously subjected to forces that vary in magnitude, location, direction, duration, frequency, variability and rate. In most cases, the body tolerates these forces well, but when loads exceed the normal physiological range- a not uncommon occurrence in elite athletes- tissues can experience overload and sustain injury. Injuries resulting from a single or a few overload episodes are called acute injuries. These injuries often happen with a violent impact, such as when a downhill skier loses control and crashes into a restraining barrier.

Where repeated loading leads to tissue damage, the injury is called an overuse or chronic injury. Calcaneal tendonitis in a long-distance runner provides chronic, overuse injury. Distinguishing acute form chronic injuries usually poses little difficulty. However, a relation between the two types sometimes exists. Chronic loading may weaken a tissue and increase its susceptibility to injury. A runner with chronic inflammation of the calcaneal tendon, may be predisposed to acute rupture of that tendon.

Torsion

A twisted structure experienced torsional loading, when the lower twists during a rapid change of direction while the foot is planted on the ground. Anatomical structures in the lower leg visit the applied torsional load. The ability of a bone to resist these applied torques depends on the bone's structural integrity. Several important principles govern a bone's torsional resistance.

1. torsion produces tensile and compressive stresses in the form of helical stress trajectories, which are maximal at the bone's surface. Excessive torsional loading can result in spiral failure along these lines.

2. shear stresses develop across the bone's cross section.

3. the stiffer the material being loaded, the harder it is to deform.

4. the larger a bone's radius, the more resistance it develops and the more difficult it is to deform.

Bending

A long, slender structure can be viewed mechanically as a beam. Forces acting perpendicular to the long axis of the beam create bending. In bending, the concave surface of the bone experience compressive stress; the convex surface of the bone is subjected to tensile stress. The maximal stresses occur at the surface of bone, with lower stresses developed away from the surface towards the midline of the bone. The bone resists the bending moment created by external forces. Greater increases in bending loads can cause the bone to fail.

Axial Loading

The simplest form of force application is uniaxial loading. In this mode, forces act along a single line, most often along the primary axis of the structure, such as when a long bone is loaded in compression or a tendon is pulled in tension by the action of its skeletal muscle. The tissue's response varies with the direction of the load. As noted earlier, biological tissues can demonstrate linear behaviour through certain loading ranges. A generalized stress-strain curve is presented. As the stress increases, the tissue's behaviour changes from its initial linear response to a non-linear region beyond,

In the real world of the athlete, forces are not always uniaxial in nature. Forces are typically multi-dimensional. The concepts of stress and strain are still applicable, but they interact across more than one dimension and thus present a more complex response.

Mechanisms of upper-extremity injuries in athletes

Most Olympic events require athletes to perform upper-extremity movements, especially overhead movements involving lifting, throwing and striking. Among these are athletic field events such as the javelin, discus, shot put, hammer throw and pole vault, as well as weight-lifting, baseball, soft-ball, volleyball and water polo. Other events such as Nordic skiing, rowing, ice hockey and swimming involve repetitive upper-extremity movements that also may predispose athletes to injury. Instability of upper-extremity joints, in particular the shoulder, and the repetitive nature of the throwing and lifting events, often lead to overuse injuries. Several such conditions and their mechanisms of injury are detailed in the following sections.

Elbow Fracture/Dislocation

In contrast to the chronic, overuse injuries just described are acute injuries caused by the rapid application of large forces. At the elbow, such injuries usually manifest as fractures or dislocations. Given the elbow's relative stability, it is no surprise that the elbow is more than three times less likely than the shoulder to suffer dislocation. Elbow joint luxation usually is accompanied by extensive soft-tissue damage that includes complete rupture or avulsion of both the ulnar and radial collateral ligaments. The elbow's bony configuration provides considerable resistance to anterior dislocation. As a result, most elbow dislocations occur posteriorly. The most common mechanics involves axial compressive forces applied to an extended or hyperextended elbow, such as would happen when someone falls onto an extended or hyperextended elbow, such as would happen when someone falls onto an extended arm. The forces in this position lever the ulna out of the trochea and rupture the capsule and ligaments, and thus allow joint dislocation.

Elbow fractures can happen to any of the three bones comprising the joint and are determined by the nature, magnitude, location and direction of the applied forces. Fracture of the distal humerus can occur in any area of the bone, including the supracondylar, intercodylar, condyle, epicodylar and articular regions. Ulhar fractures commonly involve the olecranon process, and may be caused by either direct and violent insult to the elbow joint through the forearm. Radial head fractures typically result from axial of the radius during a fall.

Musculoskeletal injuries, while an unfortunate fact of life for everyone, have special urgency for athletes, especially those committed to competing at the highest levels. Regrettably, many athletic careers have been appeared or even ended by injury. Olympic-level athletes often depend on precise upper-extremity movements for success in their sport or event. Compromised upper-extremity function caused by injury, however slight, can have profound repercussions in the athlete's performance. A clear understanding of the mechanisms of musculo-skeletal injury can aid in the effective diagnosis and treatment of the athlete, and a knowledge of injury mechanisms also may lead to better injury prevention strategies- the best injury is the one that never happens.

Valgus-Extension Mechanism

Medial epicondylitis and other injuries affecting the elbow often result from movement patterns involving throwing. Numerous studies have explored the kinematics and kinetics of the elbow during the throwing motion, which typically is divided into five phases; windup, cocking, acceleration, deceleration and flow-through. Several of these studies quantified elbow kinetics and found large and potentially injuries forces and moments. Near the end of the cocking phase, the elbow experience valgus loading as the elbow approaches terminal extension. This valgus loading is resisted by a varus torque produced by musculotendinous and particular tissues. Varus torques at this time have been estimated at between 64 and 120 Nm, with an associated joint force of about 500 N between the humerus and radius.

The coupled effect of valgus torque and elbow extension produces a valgus-extension mechanisms that can overload the joint and lead to medial elbow injuries such as epicondylitis, ulnar collateral ligament rupture, avulsion fracture and nerve damage. The valgus stress also causes compression of the lateral radio-capituopitular joint and impingement of the medial aspect of the olecranon on the olecranon fossa. Repeated impingement leads to inflammation and eventual osteophyte formation on the posteromedial aspect of he olecranon process.

In throwing, as in other dynamic movements, the highest loads occur during phases when eccentric muscle actions are required to control high-velocity motion. Repeated development of such large loads can lead to progressive tissue degeneration that culminates in failure. This process is common but not inevitable. Some athletes are able to accommodate large, repeated loads with little, if any, symptomatic response. The answer remains elusive as to why some athletes are susceptible to overload injuries while others apparently are unaffected.

Epicondylitis

Most elbow injuries result from overuse and are characterized by progressive tissue degeneration that begins with asymptomatic microtrauma and evidence of intracytoplasmic calcification, collagen fibre splitting and kinking, and abnormal fibre cross-links. Continued loading exacerbates the tissue damage and leads to symptomatic inflammation, inflexibility, and tissue weakness.

The specific dynamics of an athletic task determine whether epicodylitis affects the medial or lateral aspect of the elbow. In tennis, the lateral epoicodyle experiences injury five times as often at the medial side. Lateral epicondylitis is most commonly attributed to inflammation of the proximal attachment of the extensor carpi radialis brevis during execution of the backhand stroke.

When a player strikes the ball, forces are generated in the wrist extensor muscles. These loads are transferred through the stiffened forearm musculature to the proximal attachment on the lateral humerus. Medial epicodylists happens much less frequently in tennis players and is due largely to extreme forces developed during the forehead and service strokes when the eccentric action of wrist flexors is required to control wrist extension. In cases of both medial and lateral epicondylitis, the suspected injury mechanisms include poor stroke mechanics, off-centre ball contact with the racket, grip tightness, wrist position at contact, and racket vibration.

Lateral epicondylitis is not exclusive to tennis. Athletes in other sports that involve backhand striking movements also are susceptible a chronic pathologies of the lateral elbow. Though less common, medial epicondylitis afflicts athletes across a wide range of sports, including archery, baseball, weight-lifting, javelin, handball, swimming and racquetball.

These sports involve repetitive upper-extremity movements that predispose the athlete to overuse. The forearm muscles pose fatigue and the resulting muscle weakness leads to eccentric failure of the flexor-pronator mass. The confluence of this group's muscle attachments on the medial epicondyle is subjected to repetitive microtrauma and subsequent inflammations. Athletes affected by medial epicondylitis often are aggressive players participating at elite levels who subject their elbows to extraordinary stresses.

Elbow Injuries

The elbow provides the critical middle link in the kinetic chain of the upper extremity. It is a synovial hinge joint formed by the dual articulations of the capitulum of the humerus with the head of the radius and the trochlea of the humerus with the trochlear notch of the ulna. Normal elbow motion is limited to uniplaner flexion-extension, with forearm pronation-supination produced by concurrent rotation of the proximal and distal radio-ulnar joints. The elbow is reinforced by collateral ligament complexes on the medial and lateral aspects of the joint. Elbow flexion is controlled by concentric action of the biceps branchii, branchialis and brachioradialis, with joint extension controlled by the triceps brachii.

Before considering mechanisms of elbow injury, we note several catch-all terms used to describe elbow injuries. The most common of these is tennis elbow, a term with various meanings ranging from a general descriptor of elbow pain to a specific reference to lateral epicondylitis. As with this and other nebulous terms, we discourage their use and prefer instead to use specific clinic descriptors.

Rotatory Cuff Pathologies

Rupture of musculotendinous structures in the rotator cuff is the final step in a chain of events that has been described as an instability continuum. The progressive pathologies of instability, subluxation and impingement lead ultimately to rotator cuff tearing in some athletes. While not common in younger athletes, rotatory cuff tears can significantly affect an athlete's ability to train and perform. The loading characteristics of the rotator cuff depend on the functional demands of an athlete's sport or event.

Each sport has its own specific demands. Electromyographic data show that rapid and precise movement patterns elicit selective muscle action and periods of high muscle intensity. In spite of the unique phasic patterns particular to each throwing or striking sport motion, there is general pattern common to most. Perry described this common pattern as starting with a gentle approach to an appropriate starting position, followed by a cocking phase in which shoulder structures are tensed to provide a forceful acceleration.

Once the necessary acceleration has been accomplished, the system's muscles typically act eccentrically to decelerate the arm to avoid injurious forces. Repetitive attempts to decelerate the horizontal adduction, internal rotation, and glenohumeral distraction forces during the deceleration phase of throwing can lead to an eccentric tensile overload failure of the rotator cuff muscles, especially the supraspinatus. Repeated movements also can lead to muscle fatigue and compromised tissue integrity that contribute, in turn, to altered movement mechanics. Modifications in movement control and technique can further stress the tissues and hasten additional damage and eventual failure.

As noted, the supraspinatus is the most frequently injured muscle of the rotator cuff group and is most often associated with repeated, and often violent, overhead movement patterns. The other rotatory cuff muscles, while less susceptible to injury, are not immune to injury.

The muscles involved depend in part on the movement pattern and the task demands placed on the shoulder. Burkhart described four patterns of rotator cull kinematics associated with specific cult lesions. Type 1 lesions exhibited tears of the supraspinatus and portions of the infraspinatus, but not to an extent that disrupted essential mechanical force couples. Patients in this group had normal motion and near-normal strength.

Patients with Type-II lesions had massive teras of the superior and posterior portions of the rotator cuff. These resulted in an uncoupling of the essential force couples and led to an unstable fulcrum for glenohumeral motion. Type II patients were extremely limited and could do little more than through their shoulders.

Type III pathologies had partial tears of the subscapularis accompanying supraspinatus and major posterior cuff lesions. These injuries prevented the muscles from centering the humeral head in the glenoid fossa did led to superior humeral subluxation. Type IV lesions involved tears of the subscapularis and supraspinatus with no involvement of the posterior cuff muscles.

The complex shoulder movements required in many sports place considerable stress on the muscles of the rotatory cuff group. The throwing motion, in particular, places extraordinary loads on the shoulder. Throwing involves considerable abduction and external rotation of the arm, a position that places the rotator cuff at risk of injury, since high supraspinatus forces have been reported with the arm in the position. Those loads place the rotator cuff muscles at particular risk of injury. The role of the rotator cuff in synergistically resisting distraction of the humeral head is compromised by injury or fatigue to any of these muscles. The resulting alterations in throwing mechanics increases the likelihood of further tissue damage.

Impingement Syndrome

Much of the interest in glenohumeral impediment was stimulated by the pioneering work of Neer, who proposed an anatomical rationale and surgical treatment for chronic sub-acromical impingement syndrome. Glenohumeral impingement generally refers to arm abduction that results in the forcible pressing of supra-humeral structures, subacromial against the anterior surface of the acromion and the coracoacromial ligament that forms the coracoacromial arch. Repeated abduction impose large stresses on the capulogigamentous and musculotendinous structures of the glenohumeral joint. These stresses typically lead to tissue microtrauma, which with continued mechanical insulate can lead to tissue failure. Tissue failure then exacerbates joint instability and greater humeral movement. This, in turn, further aggravates the impingement condition. The athlete therefor is trapped in a negative feedback loop of compromised tissue integrity and joint function.

Impingement pathologies have been divided broadly into two age-related categories. Older individuals are most disposal to degenerative processes that promote bene spur formation, capsular thinning, decreased tissue perfusion, and muscle atrophy. More relevant to athletes is the second category, which includes individuals under 35 years who engage in sports involving extensive and repetitive overhead movements. Jobe and Pink proposed a classification system based on age related differences.

1. Group I injuries includes those of isolated impingement with no instability. This group typically includes older recreational athletes and only rarely includes younger athletes.

2. Group II patients exhibit instability with impingement secondary to overuse-related tissue microbrauma. This group comprise mostly young overhead athletes.

3. Group III injuries are closely associated with Group Ii pathologies common in younger athletes and are characterized by generalized ligamentous laxity and resultant shoulder instability.

4. Group IV includes injuries resulting from a traumatic event such as direct impact of a fall. Injuries in this group shoe shoulder instability without impingement.

The mechanisms of glenohumeral impingement remain controversial. The precise role of extrinsic intrinsic. Among the contributing factors are: the structural characteristics of the subacromial space 'the presence of bone spurs that focus forces on the subacromial structures and produce a functionally smaller supraspinatus outlet; degenerative processes affecting the supraspinatus; eccentric overload of the supraspinatus; muscular fatigue, compromised blood flow in regions of impingement pressure and relative tissue avascularity; and thickening of the coracoacromical ligament.

The risk factors for impingement closely parallel the

movement characteristics of sports with extensive upper-extremity involvement. These include heavy work, direct load bearing, repetitive arm movements, working with hands above shoulder height, fatigue resulting from lack of rest, and high-velocity movements.

Impingement syndrome is not restricted to the general athletic population but afflicts special population athletes as well. Wheelchair athletes, suffer a high incidence of rotator cuff impingement pathologies. Burnham et al. reported that paraplegic athletes demonstrated an imbalance of abduction/adduction strength with relative weakness of shoulder adduction. In addition, paraplegics, shoulders affected by, impingement syndrome exhibited significant weakness of adduction, external and internal rotation when compared to the uninvolved shoulders. The suggested that strengthening of shoulder adduction and internal and external rotation may be an important prevention strategy for these athletes.

Glenohumeral Instability

A joint's ability to resist laxation is directly related to its inherent structural stability. The glenohumeral joint is strengthened by ligaments and surrounding musculature including the superficial deltoid and the deeper muscles of the rotator cuff. The glenoid labrum also contributes to joint stability, to a limited degree, by increasing the surface area and deepening the fossa, and thus improving the joint's bony fit. In spite of these supporting structural elements, the glenohumeral joint remains the least stable joint is the body, a distinction substantiated by its frequent dislocation. Simply stated, what the glenohumeral joint gains in mobility, it sacrifices in stability.

At the extremes of glenohumeral joint movement, such as at the end of the cocking phase in throwing, tension in the capsulo-gigamentous structures provides resisted to dislocation. During normal ranges of motion, however, laxity in these structures precludes their involvement in stabilizing the joint to a large extent. Other mechanisms are therefore needed to ensure joint stability. These mechanisms include limited joint volume, negative intra-articular pressure, concavity compression, and scapulohumeral balance.

In a normal shoulder with an uninjured joint capsule, a small negative intracapsular pressure contributes to joint stability. While not particularly large, this negative pressure nonetheless helps stabilize the glenohumeral articulation. Concavity compression- the stability created when a convex object is pressed into a concave surface- also contributes to joint stability. The surface of the humeral head and the glenoid fossa are pressed together by multiple muscle forces.

This pressure provides greater resistance to translational movement between the surfaces. Translational resistance in the glenohumeral joint is greater in the superior inferior direction than in the anterior-posterior direction and increases with greater compressive loading. Despite the resistance provided by concavity compression, translation of the humeral head on the glenoid fossa will happen with the combined movements of glenohumeral horizontal abduction and external rotation associated with the cocking phase of throwing.

These translational movements are relevant to skill mechanics since they indicate that the glenohumeral joint does not function purely as a ball-and-socket mechanisms but allows for anterior humeral head movement during glenohumeral flexion and cross-body movements and posterior translation with extension and external rotation.

Scapulohumeral balance describes the coordinated action of muscles controlling movement of the glenohumeral joint. The muscles most immediately responsible for maintaining scapulohumeral balance are those of the rotatory cuff group. The rotatory cuff muscles are assisted by action of the deltoid, latissumus dorsi, trapezius, serratues anterior, rhomboids and levator scapulae. To maintain joint stability, the net joint reaction force created by the combined action of these muscles must remain within the glenoid fossa. When muscle forces are uncoordinated, the joint reaction force may bot be balanced within the glenoid fossa and thus contributes to joint instability. Fatigue in any of the muscles compromises the ability of the musculoskeletal system to effect proper movement mechanics.

Glenohumeral instability predictably contributes to increased potential for other pathological shoulder conditions. Kvitne and Jobe described the progressive pathology of the overhand throwing athlete along a continuum from overuse inflammatory conditions to mild joint laxity with anterior subluxation, to internal impringement syndrome, and finally to rotatory cuff tearing.

Throwing athletes require sufficient joint flexibility to achieve the joint ranges of motion required to generate high velocities. An athlete with inadequate flexibility may be advised to focus on increasing range of motion through appropriate stretching and strengthening exercises. On the other hand, repeated throwing can lead to increased joint laxity and range of motion. Brown et al., found that professional baseball pitchers exhibited 9^0 more external rotation in adduction in their dominant arm compared with the non-dominant side.

Such increases in range of motion, conceivably, could facilitate throwing performance, but more is not necessity better. Too much flexibility is detrimental since excessive stretching may enhance capsular laxity and lead to eventual shoulder instability.

Soft tissue adaptations may not be solely responsible for joint laxity. Recent evidence suggests that bony adaptations also may play a role in anterior glenohumeral instability. Pieper examined the degree of humeral retrogression in a group of male professional handball players, and found that the retrotosial angle of the humerus in a player's throwing arm was an average of 9.4° larger in the dominant side than in the non-dominant. Even more interesting form an injury perspective was the fact that in players without chronic shoulder pain, the side-to-side difference was 14.4° greater in the throwing arm. Players with chronic shoulder pain actually, showed a decrease of 5.2° of humeral retrogression in their throwing arm compared to the non-throwing arm. Piepere explained during growth to the repetitive external rotation demands of throwing practice. He concluded that Athletes who do not adapt this way seem to have more stain on their anterior capsules at less external rotation and development chronic shoulder pain because of anterior instability.

As noted previously, the glenohumeral joint is

susceptible to luxation or subluxation. In rare cases, individuals with congenitally lax shoulders may experience a traumatic glenohumeral luxations. Most cases of shoulder dislocation, however, result from traumatic forces applied directly or indirectly of the glenohumeral complex. Ninety percent of more of glenohumeal luxations happen anteriorly, usually as a result of indirect axial forces applied to an extended, abducted and externally rotated arm. These forces effectively drive the humeral-head out of its normal position in the glenoid fossa. Much less frequently, anterior glenohumeral luxations is caused by direct forces applied to the posterior aspects of the shoulder.

Mechanisms responsible for the much less common posterior luxation basically are the reverse of those causing anterior dislocation. Indirect forces transmitted through a flexed, adducted and internally rotated arm, as would be seen in landing during a forward fall, effectively during the humerus posteriorly. Posterior luxation also can result from direct trauma applied to the anterior aspect of the humerus.

Shoulder Injuries

The shoulder joint is the upper extremity's most proximal articulation and influences most movements distal to it. Efficient upper extremity throwing and lifting skills depend on adequate glenohumeral joint range of motion and neuromuscular coordination. Shoulder injury usually precludes normal movement not only of the glenohumeral joint, but also of the elbow and wrist joints, especially in multi-joint movements. Anatomically, the glenohumeral joint is formed by the articulation of the head of the humerus with the shallow glenoid fossa of the scapula. This loose fit of the humeral head within the glenoid fossa permits considerable triplanes movement, but also contributes to the least stable joint in the body.

Injury Mechanisms

Before examining the mechanics of specific musculoskeletal injuries, two terms required definition. The first is injury, defined as the damage sustained by tissues of the body. The second is mechanism, which is the fundamental physical process responsible for a given action, reaction or result.

Injury mechanisms are categorized according to mechanical concepts, tissue responses, or a combination of the two. The variety of injury types suggests a wide array of injury mechanisms. No single list or categorization system of mechanisms can adequately cover all types of injuries. Two exemplar classification systems, however, provide representative lists of injury mechanisms. Leadbetter listed contact or impact, dynamic overload, overuse, structural vulnerability, inflexibility, muscle imbalance and rapid growth as mechanisms of injury.

8

Shoulder and Arm Injuries in Sports

Upper extremity sports injuries occur less frequently than those in the lower extremity. Soft tissue injuries are most common and occur in contact sports as well as noncontact activities. Baseball, football, swimming, tennis, weightlifting, and archery are frequently associated with shoulder injuries. The type of injury varies with the activity.

Clinical history and physical examination suggest the diagnosis in many cases. Proper use arthrography, magnetic resonance imaging, and other radiographic techniques, however, is essential in confirming the diagnosis and characterizing the extent of injury.

Anatomy

The shoulder is anatomically complex, and a review of certain anatomic features is helpful in understanding how to perform imaging procedures and interpret radiographic findings.

Osteology

The clavicle is a slightly curved bone that lies ventral to the shoulder girdle. It is one of the first bones to ossify. The medial epiphysis does not unite until the end of the second decade; this should not be mistaken for a fracture. There are no secondary ossification centres distally. The clavicle articulates with the acromion distally and, rarely, with the coracoid. Medially the postal-shaped portion of the clavicle articulates with the sternum and first rib. The midportion of the clavicle is tubular, and the distal portion is relatively flat. The dorsal surface of the clavicle is roughened proximally and distally. The trapezius and deltoid muscles insert distally, and the sternocleidomastoid and pectoralis major muscles insert proximally. Inferiorly the conoid and trapezoid bands of the coracoclavicular ligament attach as the clavicle bows dorsally. The insert on the conoid tubercle and trapezoid ridge, respectively.

The scapula is dorsal to the chest well. The wing of the scapula is a large, flat, triangular bone that is almost entirely covered with muscles dorsally and ventrally. The subscapularis covers the ventral surface. Dorsally the supraspinatus takes its origin above the spine of the scapula and the infraspinatus below. The teres major and minor arise from the inferior scapula. The triceps originates from a tubercle just below the glenoid. This tubercle is usually easily visible radiographically. The supraglenoid tubercle is located just superior to the glenoid and serves as the origin of the long head of the biceps brachii. When seen in face, the glenoid lies at the junction of the scapular body with the scapular spine lying posteriorly and the coracoid anteriorly. This forms a Y with the glenoid at the junction of the scapular body with the scapular spine lying posteriorly and the coracoid anteriorly. This forms a Y with the glenoid at the junction of the limbs.

There are several secondary ossification centres that should not be confused with fractures. These include the superior glenoid, inferior glenoid, acromial, coracoid, and infra-scapular. These ossification centres usually fuse in the second decade. The glenoid ossification centres may be a source of confusion when diagnosing patients with shoulder instability.

The greater tuberosity is located laterally below the anatomic neck. This structure is seen in profile with the shoulder externally rotated. There are three facets on the greater tuberosity for insertion of three of the muscles of the rotator cuff. The insertion for the supraspinatus is most anterior, lying near the intertubercular sulcus. The infraspinatus and teres minor insert just posterior to the supraspinatus. The intertubercular sulcus lies between the greater and lesser tuberosities. Radiographically this groove normally measures about 11 mm in width and 4.6 mm in depth.

Articular Anatomy

Glenohumeral Joint

The glenohumeral joint is a ball-and-socket joint. The normally shallow glenoid cavity is much smaller than the humeral head. The cavity is deepened by a fibrocartilaginous labrum, which extends around the entire peripheral margin of the glenoid cavity.

The synovium-lined capsule attaches proximally to the glenoid labrum and extends peripherally to the anatomic neck of the humerus. The total capsules volume is nearly twice that to the humeral head. The capsule is stronger anteroirly and inferiorly and is reinforced by surrounding muscles, tendons, and ligaments. Superiorly reinforcement is achieved by the rotator cuff muscles, specifically the supraspinatus. Inferiorly there is support of the glenoid attachment by the triceps brachii, which originates from the infraglenoid tubercle. Anterior reinforcement is provided by the subscapularis tendon. Posteriorly the teres minor and infraspinatus are adjacent to the capsule. Superiorly the tendon of the long head of the biceps brachii arises from the supraglenoid tubercle and labrum. The tendon crosses the superior joint and exits through the intertubercular sulcus. This sulcus is formed by the greater and lesser tuberosities. The roof of the groove is covered by the transverse humeral ligament. The biceps tendon is covered by a synovial sheath that extends several centimetres beyond the normal capsule to about the level of the surgical neck.

Additional support is provided by four ligament complexes; the coracohumeral ligament, which arises from the coracoid to insert is the greater and lesser tuberosities; the superior glenohumeral ligament, which originates just below the coracohmeral ligament and blends with the capsule as i inserts in the lesser tuberosity; the middle glenohumeral ligament, which arises from the anterior glenoid and crosses inferiorly to the superior glenohumeral ligament to insert is the lower portion of the lesser tuberosity; and the inferior glenohumeral ligament, which arises from the anterior glenoid and inserts in the region of the surgical neck below the middle glenohumeral ligament. Stability supplied by the capsule and ligaments is augmented considerably by the rotator cuff.

There may be numerous bursae about the shoulder, but most do not communicate with the joint, and they are not always constant. The most important are the subsubscapularis bursa is situated anteriorly beneath the coracoid process and lies dorsal to the subscpaularis tendon. The infraspinatus bursa communicates with the posterior joint and lies between the capsule and the infraspinatus tendon. This is not always present.

Communication with the tendon sheath of the long head of the biceps is almost always present in the normal shoulder. A large bursa lies between the rotator cuff and acromion.

Acromioclavicular Joint

The acromioclavicular joint is a synovial joint that joins the distal clavicle and the medial portion of the acromion. An intraarticular disc is occasionally present. Both gliding and rotary motion are possible. The capsule of the joint is supported by the superior and inferior acromioclavicular ligaments; major support is derived from the coracoclavicular ligament however. Rarely, a joint is present between the coracoid and clavicle.

Sternoclavicular Joint

The medial articular portion of the clavicle forms a gliding synovial joint with the manubrium and the cartilaginous portion of the first rib. The clavicular surface is larger than the articular surface of either the manubrium or the first rib. Ligaments support includes the interclavicular ligament superiorly, the costoclavicular ligament inferiorly, and the anterior and posterior sternoclavicular ligaments. An articular disc extends from the upper clavicles to the cartilage of the first rib, dividing the joint into medial and lateral compartments.

Neurovascular Anatomy

The relationships of the neurovascular structures to the clavicle and sternoclavicular joint deserve mention.

The subclavian artery and vein pass posterior to the sternoclavicular joint. The second portion of the artery passes posterior to the scalenus anterior, which inserts into the upper portion of the first rib. The brachial plexus descends to join the vessels at this point. The auxiliary artery, a continuation of the subclavian artery, begins at the lateral margin of the first rib and extends to the distal border of the teres major. The neurovascular structures pass between the midclavicle and first rib through the axilla and along the medial aspect of the upper humerus. The major blood supply to the humerus and surrounding musculature is derived from branches of the auxiliary artery. These include the anterior and posterior humeral circumflex, clavicular, acromial, and deltoid branches from the thoracoacromial axis.

Biomechanics

The glenohumeral configuration and supporting structures of the shoulder allow uniquely complex motion. The muscles involved in glenohumeral motion are the rotator cuff, detoid, pectoralis major, latissimus dories, and teres major. Motion occurs primarily at the glenohumeral joint. Motion also occurs in the acromioclavicular and sternoclavicular joints, howcver. Glenohumeral motion is responsible for 120° of the 180° abduction arc. More than 120° of abduction requires scapular and clavicular motion. If the humerus cannot externally rotate, motion is restricted owing to impingement of the greater tuberosity on the acromion. With full abduction, the scapula is capable of rotating 60°. The major muscles producing full abduction are the deltoid, supraspinatus, trapezius, and serratus anterior.

The biomechanics of abduction have been stressed owing to common clinical problems involving the rotator cuff. This movement can be studied fluoroscopically as a part of shoulder arthorgraphy. The shoulder is also capable of flexion, extension, adduction, and rotation. The main flexors are the pectoralis major and anterior deltoid fibres, with some contribution coming from the biceps brachii. Extension is accomplished with fibres from the posterior deltoid, teres major, and latissimus dorsi. Adduction is achieved by contraction of the subscapularis, infraspinatus, teres minor, pectoralis major, latissimus dorsi, and teres major. External rotation is powered by the infraspinatus and teres minor, and internal rotation is powered by the pectoralis major, latissimus dorsi, teres major, and subscapularis.

Imaging Techniques

Routine Radiography

Numerous routine and special views have been described for evaluating the shoulder and humerus. This section discusses the routine screening evaluation plus special views that may be useful for evaluating the injured athlete.

The most useful three views for evaluating the shoulder in acute trauma include the true anteroposterior in external rotation, auxiliary, and scapular Y or Neer views. Routine views of the humerus include an AP view of the entire humorous in internal and external rotation and in certain cases transthoracic view.

The true AP view of the shoulder requires rotating the patient posteriorly 40° to see the glenohumeral joint tangentially. In the supine position the patient can be supported with a wedge or bolster. In the upright position the patient simply may be rotated. The scapular Y view of 60° anterior oblique view is obtained by elevating the shoulder or rotating the patient anteriorly 60°. This view demonstrates a Y configuration, with the Y being formed by the wing of the scapula, scapular spine, and coracoid. The glenoid is at the limbs of the Y with the humeral head centred over it. The auxiliary view generally requires abduction of the involved arm by 90°. Only mild abduction may be sufficient to allow the axillary view to be obtained. However.

On occasion it may be desirable to obtain radiographs of the bicipital groove. With the extremity in the anatomic position, the groove is positioned approximately 15° lateral to the midportion of the anterior aspect of the humeral head. Fisk suggested one method of visualizing this glove. An alternative position has the involved side elevated slightly with cushion support. The cassette is positioned above the shoulder with the hand in an anatomic position. The central beam is centered on the upper aspect of the humeral head. This view offers a projection of the length of the groove. This upper angle of the groove is better shoes in the Fisk projection.

A number of views have been developed to augment the evaluation of chronic shoulder instability. These views are designed to visualize a bony or calcific reaction, a fracture of the anterior glenoid rim, or a compression fracture of the posterior aspect of the humeral head. In the acute anterior dislocation the Hill-Sachs deformity is seen on the AP view and is usually characteristic. On occasion the humeral head can be seen to be indented posteriorly and impacted on the anterior glenoid rim, which becomes the genesis of the humeral head defect. The anterior nature of this dislocation can be confirmed with axillary or anterior oblique radiographs.

More recently, additional views have been described to identify shoulder subluxation, instability, Hill-Sachs lesions, and glenoid lesions. The apical oblique view is obtained with the patient seated or supine with the injured shoulder against the cassette and the opposite shoulder rotated 45° anteriorly. The central beam is directed 45° caudally through the shoulder with the scapula parallel to the beam because of the adducted position of he extremity. This view provides a coronal profile of the glenohumeral joint that is ideal for detection of intraarticular fractures, dislocations, instability, Hill-Sachs deformities, and glenoid injuries.

In patients who are being evaluated for recurrent anterior shoulder instability, multiple views are necessary to outline all the bone pathology because one single view does not always depict both Hill-Sachs and glenoid lesions. In these situations, the basic AP views in internal and external rotation are supplemented by a West Point axillary and a Stryker notch view. With these two additional views, it is unlikely that important findings will be missed. Fluoroscopy is also useful to obtain optimal positioning in selected cases.

Tomography

Tomography is seldom indicated in the shoulder, but it may be a useful adjunct to routine radiography and special views. This is especially true for the medial third of the clavicle and the stenoclavicular joint because thoracic contents may obscure alterations in bone structure or joint relationships. Shoulder pain is often traumatic or degenerative in origin, but small neoplasms such as an osteoid osteoma may cause difficulty in diagnosis. Radioisotope scans can localize the lesion, allowing selection of a tomographic projection to define the lesion.

Combined arthography and tomography may better define structures outlined by the contrast material.

Computed Tomography

Radiographic evaluation of the sternoclavicular joint and medial clavicular region may be difficult because of overlying structures. Computed tomography is useful for overcoming these difficulties. Scapular spine or body lesions may also be further defined with this technique.

CT has proved to be especially useful for better definition of glenoid fractures and more complex fractures because often the shoulder views are not adequate to make a decision about the need for surgery. Combined with arthrography, CT is useful for evaluating instability and glenoid labral lesions. CT arthrography is discussed more completely later.

Shoulder Arthrography

Proper choice of arthrographic technique requires an awareness of the patient's clinical problem as well as an understanding of the plain film findings. Despite the introduction of MRI, shoulder arthrography is still often used to evaluate tears of the rotator cuff and other shoulder pathology. Subtle changes in the shoulder may also be detected, especially with double-contrast techniques and by combing arthrographic techniques with CT or conventional tomography.

In a series of 552 shoulder arthrograms performed at the Mayo Clinic, 398% of patients were referred with pain and diminished range of motion. The majority of these patients were suspected to have rotator cuff lesions. An additional 19% were referred with definite clinical evidence of cuff tears. Thus 57% of the arthrograms were performed with cuff disease specifically in mind.

Knowledge of the patient's suspected problem and careful evaluation of routine radiographs can assist one in proper performance of the arthrogram and in the choice of filming sequence or CT fro the best definition of the patient's problem.

Review of plain film findings on 552 patients undergoing shoulder arthrography has provided extensive data regarding these findings. Previous reports of plain film findings in patients with rotator cuff tears describe superior subluxation of the humeral head, reversal of the normal acromial convexity, sclerosis or cystic changes in the greater tuberosity, and bony eburnation of the glenoid or humeral head inferomedially. The last finding is not a reliable indicator of rotator cuff tearing and can be seen with many chronic shoulder problems. DeSmet reported plain film abnormalities in 90.4% of 42 patients with rotator cuff tears. Our review of 552 arthrograms at the Mayo Clinic revealed 145 complete and 38 partial tears of the rotator cuff. As would be expected, changes on plain radiographs were much more common with complete chronic cuff tears. Patients with acute cuff tears less frequently demonstrate bony abnormalities on plain films.

Superior subluxation of the humeral head causes a reduction of the distance between the acromion, which is normally convex inferiorly, and the humeral head. Consistency in measurement is essential if one is to utilize this measurement properly. We measure all cases in external rotation. This measurement is virtually always greater than 1 cm in normal individuals.

Eburnation along the glenoid rim and spurring of the inferomedial aspect of the humeral head were present in 25% of patients, but this finding can also be seen with degenerative arthritis and in adhesive capsulities. Other views should also be reviewed for findings suggesting instability or previous dislocation.

Technique

With the patient in the supine position, the arm to be examined is externally rotated. A scout film is obtained to be certain that the radiographic technique is optimum. The technical quality of the films taken after injection is crucial, and preingection scout films minimize the problem of inadequate technique and the need for repeat injections.

After optimum radiographic technique is established, the patient is prepared for the procedure with a 5-minute surgical scrub and subsequent application of povidone-iodine to the skin in the area to be injected. A 5-mL syringe with 1% lidocaine and a 25-gauge needle are used to mark the site of injection. The site is chosen over the glenohumeral joint below the coracoid and approximately at the junction of the middle and distal thirds of the glenoid articular surface. A wheel is made in the skin over the joint entrance point. The soft tissues are also infiltrated with lidocaine. We err toward the medial margin of the humeral head. This ensures intraarticular positioning of the needle. The needle enters the joint of strikes the humeral head. With this technique the glenoid labrum is avoided.

The injection is made with fluoroscopic guidance to be certain that the needle is properly positioned. If it is properly positioned, the contrast material flows away from the needle around the humeral head. An extensive literature is available concerning variations in this technique.

If single-contrast technique is utilized, 6 to 10 mL of diatrizoate meglumine is injected. Low osmolality, nonionic agents are now available that may be more tolerated that ionic agents. Too much contrast material obscures detail, rendering the arthrogram less informative. With experience one can judge capsular volume early and avoid excessive amounts of contrast material. In double contrast examinations, 4 mL of contrast material and then 10 to 15 mL of air are injected, depending upon the capsule size. Again, too much contrast material defeat the purpose of a double-contrast examination. The injection must be observed fluoroscopically. If contrast material is seen to leak into the subacromial bursa during the injection, the exact site of a rotator cuff tear can be visualized.

After the injection the patient is exercised under fluoroscopic control, and any symptoms and radiographic changes are carefully noted. The relationship of the head and tuberosities to he acromion and coracoid can be examined if impingement is suspected clinically. The patient is then fluoroscopically positioned for tangential AP views of the glenohumeral joint. Films are taken in external and internal rotation. The tangential projection allows better evaluation of the articular carrilage.

Double-contrast technique is best if CT or conventional tomography is used. Lesions are less frequently obscured, and injection of air allows more time for imaging. Single contrast examinations are effective for demonstrating cuff teras and are the study of choice for adhesive capsulities. The synovium, articular cartilages, and labrum, however, are often obscured with single-contrast technique. The biceps tendon is also more difficult to evaluate. Extravasation of contrast material may be noted from the biceps tendon sheath and subscapularis bursa in normal individuals. Subtle changes, specifically tendon pathology of labral injuries, are more easily assessed with double-contrast technique.

Rotator Cuff Tears

The most common indication for shoulder arthrography is evaluation of patients with suspects tears in the rotator cuff. Many patients with rotator cuff tear have a history of trauma. The incidence is higher in patients older than 50 years of age. In our experience at the Mayo Clinic, 91% of the patients were older than 40 years of age.

The most important views are the AP views with internal and external rotation. Almost all rotator cuff tears start in or are confined to the supraspinatus tendon. With external rotation of the shoulder, this tendon is the most lateral compared with the other tendons of the rotator cuff. In rotator cuff tears, upward subluxation is most severe on this view because the amount of tendon between the humeral head and the acromion is least. In the external rotation view, the distance form the edge of the humeral head cartilage to the tendon edge as defined by the contrast material is significant. This will depict the medial to lateral length of the tear. The extent of the tear in a posterior direction, or alternatively the width of the tear, is assessed on the internal rotation view. When the shoulder is internally rotated, the infraspinatus becomes more lateral and lies under the acromion as seen on the AP view. If the upper surface and undersurface of the tendon are well outlined and complete to he tendon insertion, the tear has not extended to any degree into the infraspinatus and is thus a small or medium-sized tear. If the tendon is not well outlined on both surfaces but another tendon gap is seen, the tear has extended into the infraspinatus and is at least large in size. If the axillary view shows a normal posterior capsule pouch, the tear is large, but if the posterior pouch is also obliterated, as mentioned previously, the tear probably extends to include the posterior aspect of the infraspinatus also and is global or massive in size. Finally, an anterior oblique view should be obtained to confirm observations of the extent of the tendon tearing.

In patients with partial tears the arthorgram reveals extravasation of contrast material into a portion of the cuff without filling of the subacromial buras. Partial thickness tearing of the rotator cuff usually occurs in the supraspinatus. This can be seen as an extension of contrast material into the tendon substance but not into the bursa. If the contrast material extends past the end of the cartilage surface laterally, a portion of the tendon attachment is torn or has degenerated. These findings may be clarified by using a traction view in the upright position. Such findings also suggest that a careful evaluation is necessary because a component of the impingement syndrome related to anterior acromial osteophyte formation may well be present.

Articular Cartilage and Labral Abnormalities

Arthrography is also valuable in evaluating the articular cartilage, glenoid labrum, and synovium.

Cartilaginous lesions can be detected before they are obvious on plain films. More commonly, the arthrogram is utilized in patients with shoulder instability. Evaluation of the glenoid labrum for Bankart lesions and the humeral head for Hill-Sachs deformities may indicate dislocations. The capsule may be generous as well, indicating an additional factor contributing to the instability.

In evaluating the glenoid labrum and articular cartilage, double-contrast arthrography provides much greater detail. Care must be taken not to utilize more than 4 mL of positive contrast medium or large portions of the articular cartilage may be obscured.

We prefer both supine and prone axillary views as well as fluoroscopically positioned internal and external rotation views for the best evaluation of the labrum and articular cartilage. In patients with shoulder instability, better detail is offered by CT. Despite the introduction of MRI, many clinicians still prefer double-contrast CT. CT images are obtained after conventional images. Axial scans at 3- to 5-mm intervals are obtained with the patient supine and the arm in neutral position. With this technique the accuracy for evaluating the labrum and capsule approaches 100%. Deutsch et al reported a sensitivity of 96% and an accuracy of 86%. Callaghan et al reported a specifically of 100% for labral injuries and Hill-Sachs lesions. The ability to evaluate the biceps tendon is obvious.

Double-contrast examination with a scapular lateral view or CT is also crucial to evaluate capsule size and to detect any changes in the configuration of the anterior, posterior, and inferior recesses of the capsule. With anterior dislocations the capsule may be stripped from the glenoid, resulting in a generous anterior capsule and loss of the separation between the axillary recess and subscapularis bursa. For any significance to be attached to this, the arm must be in external rotation because it is common for this confluence to occur without instability when the arm is internally rotated. Partial or complete rotator cuff tears may also be detected in association with chronic instability. Evaluation of patients with previous trauma or surgery may be aided by an uprightweight-bearing view, which assists in determining the degree of laxity.

Loose bodies may be sufficiently ossified to be detected on routine radiographs. CT arthrography can be helpful, however, especially when the loose bodies are in such unusual locations as the biceps tendon sheath. Care must be taken not to mistake air bubbles for loose bodies. If the arthrogram is specifically requested for the detraction of osteocartilaginous fragments, single-contrast examinations may be more useful.

Bursography

We utilize bursography infrequently, and to data thc indications are still somewhat unclear. This technique may become more efficacious in the future, however, and certainly radiologists and orthopaedists should be familiar with injection or aspiration of this bursa.

The subacromial bursa is a caplike structure between the rotator cuff and the acromion with subdeltoid, subacromial, and subcoracoid portions. The normal bursa may be difficult to inject accurately.

After the radiographic study, diagnostic or therapeutic injection with bupivacaine of lidocaine and betamethasone may be performed, thus adding to the versatility of the study.

Acromioclavicular Arthrography

Radiographic approach to the acromioclavicular joint, although not as commonly employed as glenohumeral arthrography, may be of diagnostic and therapeutic value.

Patients to be studied are prepared in the usual manner with sterile technique. The joint can be entered superiorly or anteriorly after injection of local anaesthetic. Fluoroscopic guidance ensures proper positioning. One millilitre to 2 mL of diatrizoate meglumine can be injected. This amount of contrast material normally should not extend beyond the capsule. Extension of contrast material medially toward the coracoid indicates coracoclavicular ligament injury. Communication with the subacromial bursa is not uncommon in patients with chronic impingement or rotator cuff disease.

Magnetic Resonance Imaging

Techniques for MR examination of the shoulder region vary with clinical symptoms. New software and coil techniques have greatly enhanced the ability of MR examinations to evaluate patients with shoulder symptoms. A particularly important development is the ability to obtain off-axis, small field of view images in the shoulder region. This allows the patient to be examined in a more comfortable position with the arm at the side. Larger patients may need to be rotated slightly with the uninvolved arm above the head for proper positioning in the gantry. Off-axis, small-field of view images with the surface coil still represent the most optimal technique in these patients. In some cases the body coil with a smaller field of view can be utilized, but image quality is usually suboptimal.

MRI is particularly suited for evaluation of the shoulder because it is capable of detecting lesions in the rotator cuff as well as other abnormalities in the glenohumeral joint, acromioclavicular joint, and associated periarticular soft tissues.

In patients with complete rotator cuff tears it is important to identify the ends of the tendons and to calculate as closely as possible the size of the tear. Coronal and sagittal images are usually sufficient in this regard, and again T2-weighted sequences provide the best contrast distinction between the dark tendon and the high-intensity signal of the fluid between the ends of the torn tendon. In addition to demonstration of the tear, appreciation of the tendon thickness is also important. In chronic disease the tendon is often significantly thinned. Additional findings include fluid in the subacromial and subdeltoid bursae and obliteration of the normal subdeltoid fat stripe. It is not unusual in advanced disease to see communication from the glenohumeral joint through a tear into the subacromial bursa with continued extension into the acromioclavicular joint. In addition, cystic or ganglionlike lesions may appear on the dorsal aspect of the acromioclavicular joint in patients with advanced chronic rotator cuff tears. These patients may also demonstrate atrophy and retraction of the supraspinatus muscle along with the secondary osseous changes previously described.

Experience with MRI is more limited with incomplete rotator cuff tears. Incomplete tears may occur superiorly or inferiorly and are demonstrated as areas of increased signal intensity involving only a partial thickness of the tendon, usually in a linear fashion perpendicular to the course of the tendon. These findings may be difficult to differentiate from those of tendinitis. In this setting, double-contrast arthrography with weight-bearing views may still be the most effective in identifying subtle tears of the inferior surface of the tendon. Superior defects would require bursography, however, which is a more difficult technique to perform. Therefore, it is apparent that at some point MRI will also be the technique of choice in this regard.

On the basis of the work of Kneeland and Zlatkin and their colleagues, diagnostic criteria for MRI have been developed. Criteria are based on changes involving the rotator cure as well as secondary signs involving the subacromial and subdeltoid fat planes and bursae. The grading system is an follows: A normal tendon with normal signal intensity and morphology is considered grade 0. Grade 1 tendons have increased signal but normal width and morphology. A grade 2 tendon shows increased signal intensity with changes in morphology such as tendon thinning or irregularity. Grade 3 tendons have discontinuity with increased signal in the region of tendinous disruption that is best appreciated on T2-weighted images.

Burk et al compared the results of arthrography, MRI, and ultrasound in a group of 38 patients referred for suspected rotator cuff tears. Both MRI and double-contrast arthrography demonstrated sensitivities of 92% and specification of 100% for normal cuffs. Diagnosis of cuff tears was equal with both techniques. Ultrasound was 63% sensitive for diagnosis of cuff tears and demonstrated as specificity of only 50% for intact rotator cuffs. Others have reported ultrasound to have an accuracy of 87% to 94% for diagnosis of rotator cuff tears; importantly, the negative predictive value of ultrasonography was 95%. In the operated group, however, the specificity of ultrasound was only 73% compared to 100% for arthrography.

Arthrography is an accurate but invasive technique for diagnosis of rotator cuff tears, but it is of little value in evaluating impingement. Ultrasound is accurate in some physicians' hands but has not achieved the wide acceptance of MRI or arthrography because of the experience required by examiners and its difficulty in achieving acceptance in the orthopaedic community. Physicians not involved in performing and interpreting ultrasound find the image difficult to evaluate. MRI is noninvasive and provides a method of screening for many osseous and soft tissue abnormalities. Although refinements are still in progress, it appears to be the noninvasive technique of choice for evaluating impingement and rotator cuff pathology.

Imaging of Capsular Abnormalities

The capsular structures of the shoulder consist of the synovial membranes, the capsule, the associated glenohumeral ligaments, the glenoid labrum, and associated bursae and recesses. The subscapularis muscle and tendon are also closely applied to the anterior capsule. Imaging of the shoulder capsule has conventionally been accomplished with either conventional or CT arthrography. Contrast arthrography provides valuable information regarding the size and intergrity of the capsule and also allows intraarticular injections of anaesthetic and/or a combination of anaesthetic and steroid compounds to treat and diagnose certain shoulder disorders.

Capsular volume is difficult to evaluate with noncontrast MRI because the degree of distention of the capsule cannot be evaluated unless contrast material of some type is injected. Recently, gadolinium-DTPA has been advocated as an MR arthrography contrast agent. To date, however, there has not been enough significant experience to understand clearly its implications in MRI of the shoulder. Certainly fluoroscopically monitored injections of contrast material are much more efficacious than MR arthrography at this point. Therefore, patients who are being evaluated for subtle changes in the synovial lining or for changes in capsular volume such as adhesive capsulities are still studied to better advantage with conventional arthrography or arthrography combined with CT or conventional tomography.

Disruption of the shoulder capsule can be detectable by arthrography or MRI. Loss of integrity of the capsule or its adjacent or associated ligaments can be identified on MRI as poorly defined areas of increased signal intensity adjacent to the capsule on T-2 weighted sequences. Capsular lesions are most easily evaluated in the axial and coronal planes.

Recurrent shoulder dislocations are a common problem in orthopaedic practice. Originally, it was believed that the. Bankart lesion was the main lesion causing recurrent anterior dislocation. More recently the entire anterior capsule mechanism has been implicated. Type 2 and 3 capsular insertions are more often associated with instability.

Fractures, Dislocations, and Osseous Injuries

Fractures of the Proximal Humerus

Fractures of the proximal humerus usually occur

in older patients. If one considers all fractures, about 5% involve the proximal humerus. In older patients, the fracture most often occurs after minor trauma, such as a fall. In younger individuals and athletes, the skeletal strengths greater than that provided by ligaments, so that dislocations usually occur instead of fractures. When fractures occur in this age group, they usually result from a fall with the elbow flexed and wrist dorsiflexed. Eighty per cent of humeral fractures in children involve the proximal epiphysis.

Fractures of the proximal humerus tend to follow the phy-seal lines that divide the humerus into four parts: the humeral head, lesser tuberosity, greater tuberosity, and shaft. Neer proposed the most widely accepted classification for adult fractures of the proximal humerus. This classification is based on the number of fragments and the degree of displacement or angular deformity. If there is 1 cm of displacement between the fragments of greater than 45° of angular malposition, the fragment is considered displaced.

The majority of proximal humeral fractures are undisplaced. Fractures most commonly involve the surgical neck. The rotator cuff, capsule, and periosteum assist in maintaining the position of the fragments. A two-part fracture indicates that one fragment is displaced more than 1 cm or angulated more than 45°. Three-part fractures have two displaced or angulated fragments. With four-part fractures, all fragments are displaced. Isolated fractures of the tuberosities are rare unless there is an associated dislocation.

Accurate radiographic evaluation of the shoulder can be obtained with the shoulder trauma series. AP and lateral views are usually adequate to define humeral shaft fractures. Proper classification requires experience. Because the majority of fractures are undisplaced, it is not surprising that interobserver errors are higher with three-and four-part fractures. CT is useful to ensure proper classification and for accurate assessment of fragment position before therapy.

Glenohumeral Dislocations

Dislocations of the glenohumeral joint occur more frequently than dislocations at nay other articulation. They account for 50% of all dislocations. Most dislocattions are anterior. Posterior dislocations occur in 2.0% to 4.3% of patients, and superior and inferior dislocations are rare.

Anterior Dislocations

Most anterior dislocations are due to trauma, usually resulting form a fall with the arm in abduction and external rotation. Rarely, the dislocation is due to direct posterolateral trauma. In adolescence, dislocations in boys outnumber those in girls by 5:1. As the humeral head dislocates, it is forced anteriorly and inferiorly against the capsule, glenohumeral ligaments, and subscapulatris. These structures gelnohumeral ligaments, and subscapularis. These structures provide the majority of the shoulder's anterior stability. The posterolateral aspect of the humeral head comes in contact with the glenoid rim, which may result in an associated impaction fracture. This was described by Hill and Sachs and bears their name, the Hill-Sachs deformity. This lesion occurs in 67% to 76% of cases. Associated lesions of the anteroinferior glenoid rim reportedly occur less frequently, appearing in approximately 50% of cases.

After closed reduction, the radiographic trauma series, except for the axillary view, should be repeated. The radiographs must be carefully studied to ensure adequate reduction and to exclude associated fractures. For example, if the anterior dislocation results in the humeral head lying medial to the coracoid, reduction may be more difficult. Interruption of the tendon of the long head to the biceps may occur with this type of dislocation, making reduction difficult or impossible. Displacement of the biceps tendon should also be considered in dislocations with large greater tuberosity fractures because the bicipital groove may be involved. Fractures of the greater tuberosity occur in up to 15% of anterior dislocations. Rarely, coracoid fractures occur with anterior dislocation.

Posterior Dislocations

Only about 2.0% to 4.3% of shoulder dislocations are posterior. In sports, the injury usually occurs during falls with the arm adducted and internally rotated or with direct rauma to the anterior shoulder.

Clinically, the patient's arm may be held in slight abduction and internal rotation. External rotation in blocked. The diagnosis is missed clinically in many patients.

The injury may be easily overlooked on the conventional AP view. There are, however, several signs present:

- The humeral head is fixed in internal rotation
- The joints may appear abnormally widened or narrowed.
- The usual half-moon overlap of the humeral head and glenoid may be absent or distorted.

- A trough line may appear in the humeral head, representing a compression fracture of the anterior aspect of the humeral head.
- There may be an associated fracture of the lesser tuberosity.

Superior and Inferior Dislocations

Superior and inferior dislocations are rare. Superior dislocations overlie the acromion or clavicle on the AP view. This dislocation is usually due to a severe upward force on the adducted arm. With luxatio erecta, the humerus becomes parallel to the spine of the scapula, and the arm is abducted. Downy et al reported this type of dislocation in 0.5% of all dislocations. This injury is due to force on the flexed arm. As a result, the humeral head is forced downward. Inferior subluxation may be associated with humeral fractures, glenoid fractures, capsular tears, or brachial plexus injury. These types of dislocations can usually be managed initially with closed reduction, but more injuries and rotator cuff tears may be present.

Complications of Glenohumeral Dislocations

Complications of glenohumeral dislocations and fracture-dislocations are more common than complications of proximal humeral fractures. Associated fractures and recurrent dislocations are the most common problems. Other associated fractures include those of the greater tuberosity and, less frequently, the coracoid as well as lesser tuberosity of subscapularis anteriorly.

Acromioclavicular dislocations

Dislocations of the acromioclavicular joint occur less commonly than glenohumeral dislocations. The mechanism of injury is usually a fall in which force is directed to the point of the shoulder. Dislocations due to indirect forces directed superiorly through the humeral head have also been reported.

Treatment of most type I and II injuries is successful with closed methods. Occasionally, closed excision is necessary. Internal fixation is more often necessary with type III adult injuries.

Adjacent fractures can accompany acromioclavicular dislocation. In our experience at the Mayo Clinic, the coracoid and clavicle are fractured most frequently. Intraarticular acromial fractures may also occur.

Sternoclavicular Dislocations

Dislocations of the sternoclavicuar joint are uncommon. Dislocation usually results from indirect trauma to the shoulder. Posterolateral forces transmitted medially cause anterior dislocation. Direct anterior trauma can occur in sports such as football. This causes posterior dislocation. Anteriro dislocations occur much more frequently than posterior dislocations. Anterior dislocations may be easily palpable. Posterior dislocations can be more difficult to diagnose clinically owing to swelling. Early diagnosis is necessary because reduction after 48 hours is difficult. In addition, posterior dislocations may be potentially fatal injuries because of involvement of the trachea and great vessels.

Clavicle Fractures

Clavicle fractures are common, especially in children. The injury usually is caused by a fall on the outstretched hand. The lateral force directed through the should results in fracture of the midclavicle less frequently direct trauma to the clavicle or shoulder results in fracture.

Fractures of the middle third of the clavicle are most common Allman classified clavicle fractures anatomically. Group I fractures involve the middle third of the clavicle. Displacement of these fractures is common. The sternocleidomastoid elevates the proximal fragment, and the weight of the arm tends to lower the distal fragment. This results in a superior tended radiographic appearance. Group II fractures involve the distal clavicle. These fractures make up 15% of clavicle fractures. Group III fractures involve the medial clavicle.

Radiographic evaluation of the middle and distal clavicle is not difficult. AP or oblique views of the clavicle, with the tube angled 15° or more to the head, will allow good visualization of the middle and sital clavicle. The angulation projects the clavicle above the chest. A coned-down 15° angled view is best to overcome the problem of overpenetrating the acromioclavicular joint. Subtle midclavicle fractures may be overlooked. If symptoms dictate, a 40° cephalad angle may make detection less difficult. Evaluation of the proximal clavicle is more difficult. Forty-degree angled views and oblique views are usually adequate if the fracture is displaced. In selected cases, especially undisplaced fractures, CT may be necessary.

Most clavicle fractures can be treated with closed reduction and shoulder support. Group II fractures of the distal clavicle may require internal fixation. Resection of the distal clavicle may be required in patients with persistent symptoms.

Significant complications are less common with clavicle fracture is displaced. In selected cases, especially undisplaced fractures, CT may be necessary.

Most clavicle fractures can be treated with closed reduction and shoulder support. Group II fractures of the distal clavicle may require internal fixation. Resection of the distal clavicle may be required in patients with persistent symptoms.

Significant complications are less common with clavicle fractures than with glenohumeral fracture-dislocations. Malunion of midclavicle fractures or excessive callus formation does occur. This may result in compression of the adjacent neurovascular structures between the clavicle and first rib.

Nounnion occurs on only 1% to 2% of cases. Osteoarthritis may occur after intraarticular fracture. This is more common at the acromioclavicular joint. Posttraumatic osteolysis may be seen in the distal clavicle. Patients present with continued pain and weakness after trauma. Erosive changes develop on the distal clavicle; these are visible on the radiograph. Involvement may progress to the level of the coracolavicular ligaments. Changes may be due to synovial hyperplasia, but this is uncertain. After treatment with immobilization some degree of bone healing occurs, although the joint often remains widened.

Scapular Fractures

Fractures of the scapula are uncommon . Injury to the body of the scapula is caused by direct force. The scapula is well protected by an envelope of muscles. There fore, considerable force is required to cause the fracture. And displacement of body fractures is usually not significant. Fractures of the body of the scapula are rare in athletes.

Fractures of the body may extend to the glenoid articular surface. Most commonly, glenoid fractures are associated with dislocations. Varriale and Adler, however, have described glenoid fractures that are not associated with dislocation. Fractures may be undisplaced, displaced, or bursting. Detection of glenoid fractures is crucial because, If displaced, they lead to traumatic arthritis. Scapular Y, West Point, and axillary views are most useful in demonstrating these fractures. Avulsion fractures of the infraglenoid tubercle are due to forceful triceps contraction. This fracture may also lead to recurrent dislocation, especially if a portion of the rim is involved.

Fractures of the acromion usually are due to a direct blow from above. Stress fractures, however, may also occur in association with dislocations and rotator cuff tears. Radiographic diagnosis is not difficult in most cases. The axillary and Y views are particularly useful in the diagnosis of subtle acromial fractures.

Fractures of the coracoid process may be due to direct trauma or avulsion. Muscular origins of the coracoid include the coracobrachialis, short head of the biceps, and pectoralis minor. Most fractures occur at the base. Displacement is usually prevented by ligament attachment.

Repeated trauma in trapshooters may result in a coracoid stress furcate. Radiographic evaluation of coracoid fractures should include the scapular Y view and the axillary view. In addition, weight-bearing views should be considered. Fractures of the coracoid are associated with acromioclavicular dislocation.

Miscellaneous Osseous Conditions

Several additional conditions have been described that result in shoulder pain. Posttraumatic osteologist of the clavicle was mentioned above.

Osteochondritis dissecans is most common in the knee and then in the ankle, hip, and elbow. Rarely, the condition may also affect the glenoid. The lesion is not difficult to identify if it is located away from the inferior labrum. In this setting, confusion with a Bankart lesion may occur. True AP and auxiliary views are most useful. CT or MRI, however, is most useful for staging and complete evaluation of this unusual lesion.

Little league shoulder is a condition described in young baseball pitchers. The condition is due to repeated trauma and was believed to be a growth plate fractures. Barnett prefers the term proximal humeral epiphyseolysis. The involved epipysis is irregular and widened; these changes are similar to those noted with slipped capital femoral epiphysis. Changes are usually readily apparent on AP views of the shoulder. Patients present with pain when throwing. Healing occurs with rest. The condition must be differentiated from impingement syndrome.

Blocker's exostosis is due to contusion or repetitive trauma to the region of the deltoid insertion on the humerus. Trauma to this region is common in offensive linemen and others involved in blocking during football plays. Repeated trauma can lead to painful periostitis and adjacent soft tissue injury. If the area is not properly protected, an organized exostosis that extends anterolaterly from the humerus may occur. Conservative therapy with protection of the area during the early stages is the best method of therapy.

Soft Tissue Trauma

Certain aspects of soft tissue trauma have been discussed above. Soft tissue injuries are common in athletes, however, and certain conditions deserve further attention, specifically as they apply to imaging evaluation.

Rotator Cuff and Capsular Injuries

Shoulder injuries are particularly common in tennis, swimming, and throwing sports such as base ball. Forty percent to 80% of competitive swimmers develop shoulder symptoms. Symptoms are most common in swimmers after 6 to 8 years of competition. The butterfly, freestyle, and backstroke techniques are implicated most frequently.

In addition, up to 65% of baseball players develop rotator cuff injuries.

The arm and shoulder in these sports have similar motions. The arm is abducted and externally rotated, stretching the anterior capsules and muscles with maximal contraction posteriorly. When the player is striking a tennis ball or throwing a ball, the shoulder moves from abduction and external rotation into forward flexion and internal rotation. When the arm is abducted and externally rotated, the cuff and subacromial bursa are impinged between the humerus and acromion. In addition to impingement, biceps tendinitis and instability may be present. The latter is probably due to repetitive capsular stretching.. Rotator cuff tears and labral injuries are uncommon in young athletes.

Athletes engaged in the above activities usually present with shoulder pain. Pain may be generalized, but more often the symptoms are anterior or lateral.

Symptoms may be related to impingement and/or associated biceps tendinitis.

The arch of the shoulder is formed by the clavicle, acromioclavicular joint, anterior acromion, and coracoacromial ligament. The subacromial bursa allows smooth motion between the arch and the humeral head. Abnormalities in the structures of this arch may lead to impingement. Three stages of impingement have been described. Stage 1 changes occur in young athletes and include oedema and hemorrhage. These changes occur most commonly in the critical zone just medial to the supraspinatus insertion. Stage 2 changes occur in older athletes after years of repetitive microtrauma. Fibrosis of the subacromial bursa, thick ending of the coracoacromial ligament, and subtle acromial or greater tuberosity changes may be evident. Stage 3 changes typically occur in patients 40 years old or older. Further degeneration and rotator cuff tears occur.

Related conditions such as instability may have similar presentations. Athletes may describe a dead arm, which is probably related to repetitive capsular stretching.

A related condition, tennis shoulder, is a postural change in the exercised extremely .and results in drooping of the shoulder and scoliotic changes in the thoracic spine. This condition is due to repetitive stretching of the trapezius, levator scapulae, and rhomoboideus minor and major, which allows the shoulder to drop. There is also an increase in the muscle and osseous mass of the extremity, which contributes to the postural change.

Imaging of athletes with shoulder pain should ideally identify abnormalities in bone, muscle, ligaments, and tendons. Multiple techniques have been used to identify capsular abnormalities and rotator cuff injuries. Routine radiographs provide useful secondary signs of cuff and capsular abnormalities. Superior subluxation of the humeral head reducing the humeroacomial distance to less than 7 mm indicates rotator cuff injury. Changes in the acromion, acromioclavicular joint, and greater tuberosity are also useful. Hypertrophic change in the acromioclavicular joint, subacromial sclerosis and spur for nation, and erosions or sclerosis of the greater tuberosity are useful findings. Special views described earlier, including the apical oblique view, fluoroscopy, and the scapular Y view, are useful in this regard.

Arthorgraphy was once the gold standard for evaluating the rotator cuff and capsule. Although MRI has gained wide acceptance, arthrography, especially with CT, is still a valuable technique. Partial and complete tears can be accurately diagnosed with routine arthrography. On multiple views of CT the capsule volume and other abnormalities can also be identified. Sonography is also useful for evaluating the rotator cuff, but it is less useful as an overall screening technique for shoulder disorders.

MRI, as previously discussed, is an effective technique for evaluating patients with suspected impigement, rotator cuff tears, and capsular abnormalities. Utilization of T2 weighted sequence in the coronal, sagittal, and axial planes provides valuable information regarding the cuff, capsule, arch of the shoulder, and surrounding soft tissues.

Changes suggesting cuff disease and impingement on routine films or bursography can be even more accurately assessed with MRI. Bone articular, and soft tissue changes can all be identified. Changes in the acromion and the acromioclavicular and coracoacromial ligaments are obvious. The shape of the acromion may be significant; it may be flat, gently curved, or hooked anteriorly. The last is associated with rotator cuff disease.

Signal intensity changes and variations in thickness are most useful in assessment of the rotator cuff. The double-echo T2-weighted spin-echo sequence is most useful, but gradient-echo techniques may also be used. Chronic cuff disease or tendintis manifests as slight variation in thickness with mild increased signal intensity on the first echo and little or no increase in signal intensity on the second echo. Partial tears are seen as areas of increasing intensity on the second echo that do not fully involve the tendon. The most specific sign of a full thickness tear is fluid or high signal with no cuff evident. The axial views is also useful when small cuff tears are present and involve areas other than the supraspinatus. Secondary signs of rotator cuff tears include supraspinatus muscle retraction, irregularity of the superior margin of the cuff, thinning, indistinct subdeltoid flat plane, and fluid in the subacromial bursa. The last can be seen with bursitis alone. Specificity and sensitivity of MRI in evaluating cuff disease are both approximately 90%.

Biceps Injuries

Biceps injury or tendinitis is frequently associated with rotator cuff disease. The biceps tendon passes adjacent to the superior labrum as it crosses the joint and enters the biceps groove between the greater and lesser tuberositis. Biceps tendon injuries include inflammation or overuse syndromes, subluxation, dislocation, and rupture. Injuries occur most frequently swimmers and throwing athletes.

Patients usually present with anterior shoulder pain. Pain may also be more generalized because it is frequently associated with impingement. These symptoms may mask underlying instability. Therefore, imaging should provide information about stability, impingement, and the biceps tendon.

9

Foot and Ankle Injuries in Sports

Fifty-five per cent to 90% of sports injuries involve the lower extremity, most commonly the knee, foot, and ankle. The majority of foot and ankle injuries are related to running, jumping, or cutting manoeuvres.

Acute foot and ankle injuries account for 10% of emergency department visits. Overuse injuries are also common, however, and most often are not seen in an emergency setting.

Overuse syndromes in the foot account for 50% of injuries. The highest incidence in the series reported by Garrick and Requa occurred in volleyball; running and tennis, racquetball, and gymnastics has the next highest incidence rates. Sprains do occur in the foot, but they account for less than 7% of foot injuries.

Knowledge of the anatomy and clinical data are essential requirements for optimal imaging of the foot and ankle. Therefore, these aspects of foot and ankle injuries are emphasized along with specific imaging techniques.

Anatomy

Basic osseous and soft tissue anatomy is discussed here.

Osseous and Ligamentous Anatomy of the Ankle

The ankle is formed by three bones: The tibia, and

fibula, and the talus. The tibia is the second longest bone in the skeleton. It is expanded proximally and distally. The body of the tibia has three surfaces: anterior, medial, and posterior. The anterior surface ends in the medial mellifluous. The medial margin is subcutaneous. The interosseous membrane attaches to the lateral margin.

The anterior surface of the tibia is smooth except at the anteroinferior margin, where it is more irregular at the site for attachment of the anterior ankle capsule. The posterior tibia has grooves for the flexor hallucis longus and flexor digitorum longus and tibialis posterior tendons. The lateral surface articulates with the fibula. This articular surface is bounded anteriorly and posteriorly by ridges for insertion of the anterior and posterior distil tibiofibular ligaments. The strong medial extension articulates with the talus and forms the medial portion of the ankle mortise.

The fibula is this and flat and does not have a direct weightbearing surface. The lateral malleolus is the expanded distal portion of the fibula. The fibula is irregular along its medial margin at the point of attachment for the interosseous ligament. Hyaline carilage covers the articular surface on the inferomedial aspect. There are irregular areas anteriorly and posteriorly for insertions of the tibiofibular ligament. The fibula is more posterior than the medical malleolus, and its distal extent is below the level of the medical malleolar tip. Thus an angle of about 8° is formed by a line drawn from the tips of the malleoli. The posterior position of the lateral malleolus results in an angle of 20° between the malleoli in the axial plane. For this reason the mortise view of the ankle is taken with the foot internally rotated approximately 20°.

The hyaline cartilage trochlear surface of the talus

is usually 2 to 3 mm wider anteriorly than posteriorly. It articulares with the weight-bearing surface of the tibia and the medial and lateral malleoli. Thus the ankle mortise is formed by the tibial and fibular components of the ankle, which roofs the talus. The tibial portion of the mortise is termed the plafond. Forces on the talus that result in position changes of this structure in the mortise are responsible for many osseous and/or ligamentous ankle injuries.

The deltiod ligament provides medial stability. This ligament is strong, triangular-shaped group of fibres with its apex at the medial maleolus. The ligament fans out as it progresses inferiorly and divides into superficial and deep fibres. The superficial fibres insert in the navicular tuberosity. Progressing posteriorly, the remaining superficial fibres insert in the sustentaculum tali and the talus. The deep fibres attach to the medial surface of the talus. The deltoid ligament prevents excessive abduction and eversion of the ankle and subtalar joints. In addition, eversion, pronation, and anterior displacement of the talus are restricted.

Foot Anatomy

For purposes of discussion, the foot can be divided into three segments: the hindfoot, midfoot, and forefoot. Three longitudinal columns have also been described. The medial column consists of the calcaneus, talus, navicular, medial and intermediate cuneiforms, and first and second metatarsals and phalanges. The middle column consists of the lateral cuneiform and the third metatarsal and phalanx. The lateral column is made up of the hindfoot and the fourth and fifth metatarsals with their phalanges. All articulations are synovial joints supported by strong plantar and weaker dorsal ligaments.

Hindfoot

The hindfoot includes the talus and calcaneus. The talus is the second largest of the tarsal bones and articulates with the tibia, medial and lateral malleoli, and calcaneus inferiorly. The talar head artisculates with the navicular.

Superiorly the trochlea articulates with the tibia and malleoli. It is covered with hyaline cartilage and makes up the upper portion of the body of the talus. There are three articular facets on the inferior surface of the talus. The anterior and posterior facets articulate with similarly named calcaneal articular facet. The middle facet articulates with the sustentaculum tali. The talar sulus lies between the middle and anterior facets. The structure with its calcaneal counterpart forms the tarsal sinu, which contains the interosseous talocalcaneal ligament. The head of the talus articulates with the navicular.

Several osseous growths have been described on the talus. These are usually of no clinical significance. A normal ridge is present distal to the trochlear surface on the dorsolateral aspect of the talus. This can be seen on the lateral view of the ankle and should not be confused with pathology. This ridge is the site of attachment of the dorsal talonavicular ligament and anterior tibviotalar joint capsule. Therefore, hypertrophy can occur in patients engaged in activities that require extremes of planter flexion. The posterior aspect of the talus contains an oblique groove for the flexor hallucis longus tendon.

The calcaneus, which is the largest tarsal bone, contains three superior articular facets. The middle, most medial facet is on the sustentaculum tali. The calcaneal sulcus lies between the middle and anterior facets and forms the floor of the tarsal canal. This canal has an oblique course and measures 10 to 15 mm is height, 3 to 5 mm in width, and 15 to 20 mm in length. The distal or plantar surface of the calcaneus contains two grooves. The lateral groove. The lateral groove is for the peroneus longus tendon. More medially, the flexor hallucis longus runs in the groove beneath the sustentaculum tali.

Midfoot

The remaining tarsal bones make up the midfoot. These include the cubiod, the navicular, and three cuneiforms.

The cuboid articulates with the calcaneus proximally and with the fourth and fifth metatarsals distally. Dorsally the cuboid is roughened at the points of ligament attachment. On the planter surface the cuboid contains a groove for the peroneus longus tendon. The medial cuboid surface contains a facet font articulation with the lateral cuneiform.

The navicular is on the medial side of the foot anterior to the talus. It articulates proximally with the talus, anteriorly with the cuneiforms, and occasionally laterally with the cuboid.

The spring ligament is contiguous with the deltoid ligament of the ankle. It extends from the calcaneus to the navicular tuberosity. The cubonavicular ligament runs dorsally from the cuboid to the navicular. Proximally the bifurcate ligament originates on the anterosuperior calcaneus and sends medial fibres to the lateral navicular and lateral fibres to the cuboid. The calcaneonavicular ligament is on the plantar aspect of the capsule.

There are three cuneiform bones located distal to the navicular and medial to the cuboid. The medial cuneiform is the largest and articulates with the navicular proximally, the intermediate cuneiform laterally, and the first and second metatarsal distally. The intermediate cuneiform is the smallest cuneiform and lies between the medial and lateral cuneiforms. It articulates with the latter bones, the navicular, and the second metatarsal. The lateral cuneiform lies between the intermediate cuneiform and the cuboid, articulating with both. It also articulates with the navicular and the second through fourth metatarsals.

The five metatarsals articulate proximally with the tarsal bones described above, and each, except the first, typically has three phalanges distally. The metatarsals have a similar configuration except that the first is broader from the proximal articular surface distally to its head. The fifth metatarsal has a broad base compared to the second through fourth metatarsals.

Arches of the Foot

There are three arches in the foot: one transverse and two longitudinal. The lateral longitudinal arch is formed by the calcanesus, cuboid, and fourth and fifth metatarsals. In a patient with normal gait, this arch normally receives the weight of the body before the medial longitudinal arch. The peroneus longus tendon runs through the midpoint of this arch. The medial longitudinal arch is formed by the calcaneus, talus, navicular, cuneiforms, and first through third metatarsals. The vertical height of the medial arch is greater than that of the lateral arch. The apex of the arch is more posterior, being located at the calcaneotalonavicular junction. The posterior tibial tendon inserts on the navicular and sends plantar fibres below the arch, adding additional support.

The transverse arch is completed when the feet are

adjacent, so that the two medial longitudinal arches are approximated. Thus the bases of the metatarsals and midtarsal bones form the arch with support from the peroneus longus and posterior tibial tendons.

Normal Variants

There are many anatomical variants that can mimic more serious pathologic conditions. These changes arc most common in the metaphyseal and epihyseal areas adjacent to the growth plates. Occassionally small ossification centres are evident adjacent to he growth plates, simulating fractures. Ossicles are also commonly noted near the medial and lateral malleoli. These frequently cause confusion in diagnosing patients with recent injury. They occur medially in 17% to 14% of girls and up to 47% of boys. Most are bilateral, and they are commonly seen from 6 to 12 years. Normal variants are also common in the tarsal bones.

The secondary ossification centre of the talus is located posteriorly. It appears at 8 to 11 years of age and normally fuses at 16 to 20 years of age. This somewhat controversial ossification centre is the posterior part of the talar tubercle and is located lateral to the flexor hallucis longus tendon. If this centre does not fuse to the talus, it is called the so trigonum tarsi and is frequently mistaken for a fracture. In forced plantar the ossicle can separate, or fracture can occur in the fused centre.

Another common finding is the accessory navicular, or as tibial externum. This lies in the posterior tibial tendon just proximal to the medial margin of the navicular. This ossicle may affect tendon function, especially during puberty when growth is accelerated. Resection may be required to relieve the painful symptoms. The os supranaviculatre is located at the proximal dorsal margin of the navicular distal to the joint space. This is more distal than the os supratalare, which would be proximal to the talonavicular joint. The most frequently noted ossicles in the foot are summarized in.

Soft Tissue Anatomy

The muscles of the calf are divided into anterior, posterior, and lateral compartments. Because of their action on the foot and ankle, a brief review of anatomy and function is in indicated.

The muscles of the deep posterior compartment also act on the foot and ankle except for the populates, which serves as a flexor of the knee. The flexor hallucis longus serves as a flexor of the great toe, and the flexor digitorum longus assists in plantar flexing the foot and serves as a flexor of the lateral four toes. The tibialis posterior is the deepest muscle of the posterior compartment. Its tendon passes anterior to the flexor digitorum under the flexor retinaculum to insert on the navicular and tarsal bones. This muscle aids in adduction, inversion, and plantar flexion. Neurovascular supply to the posterior muscles is via the tibial nerve and posterior tibial artery.

The personas longus and brevis are the muscles of the lateral compartment. The tendons enter a common sheath above the ankle and pass posterior to the lateral malleolus and deep to the peroneal retinacula. On the tateral surface of the foot the peroneus brevis inserts on the lateral surface of the foot the peroneus brevis inserts on the fifth metatarsal base. The peroneus longus passes under the foot to insert on the medial cuneiform and first metatarsal base. Both muscles assist in eversion and plantar flexion of the foot.

The anterior compartment comprises the extensor digitorum longus, peroneus tertius, extensor hallucis longus, and tibialis anterior. The extensor digitorum longus aids in dorsiflextion of the foot and lateral four toes. The extensor hallucis longus serves mainly for dorsiflextion of the great toe. The tibialis anterior inserts at the midfoot and aids in dorsiflexion and inversion of the foot. Neurovascular supply to the anterior and lateral compartments is via the peroneal nerve and anterior tibial and peroneal arteries.

The musculature of the foot is complex. A complete discussion of origins and insertions is beyond the scope of this text. Certain functional aspects will be discussed, but the reader is referred to other texts of a more in-depth discussion. The muscles of the foot are divided into four layers. The superficial muscles include the abductor hallucis, flexor digitorum brevis and abductor digit minimi. The former is a weak abductor of the great toe and is supplied by the medial plantar artery and nerve. The centrally located flexor digitorum brevis has the same neurovascular supply. It serves as a flexor of the lateral four toes. The abductor digit minimi is a flexor and abductor of the fifth toe.

The second layer of muscles includes the quadratus plantae, lumbrical muscles, and tendons of the flexor hallucis longus and flexor digitiorum longus. These muscles assist in flexion of the toes. Neurovascular supply is via both medial and lateral plantar artery and nerve branches.

The third layer includes the flexor hallucis brevis, adductor hallucis, and flexor digiti minimi brevis. The flexor hallucis aids in flexion of the great toe, and the adductor hallucis serves as an adductor of the great toe. The flexor digiti minimi flexes the small toe.

The fourth and deepest muscle layer includes the three painter and four dorsal interosseous muscles. The dorsal interossei act as abductors and the plantar interossei as adductors of the foot.

The extensor digitorum brevis is the dorsal muscle of the foot. The muscle is a corsiflexor of the great toe and second through fourth toes.

Common Terms

Terms used to describe the movements in the foot and ankle are often misused. This results in some confusion when descriptive terms such as supination, eversion, pronation, and the like are used. Definitions of these commonly used terms are listed below as they apply during physiologic motion of the foot and ankle.

- Plantar flexion: The hinge motion at the tibiolalar joint allows the foot to plantar flex. Several other motions and position changes occur with plantar flexion. During plantar flexion the gastrocnemius muscle pulls the calcaneus upward, which shifts the calcaneus into a slight varus position. The head of the talus turns in and downward during plantar flexion, which causes the foot to move inward.
- Dorsiflexion: The hinge motion of the ankle allows the foot to be elevated or dorsiflexed. The gastrocnemius muscle is relaxed, and the heel shifts into a valgus position. The talus turns upward and outward, so that the foot also furns outward during dorsiflexion.
- Inversion: During inversion the sole of the foot is turned inward. In the European literature the terms supination and adduction are often used interchangeably with inversion. The foot tends to dorsiflex slightly during inversion.
- Eversion: During eversion the sole of the foot is

turned outward. The terms pronation and abduction have been used interchangeably with eversion. The foot tends to plantar flex slightly during eversion.

- Adduction: By definition, adduction means movement of a part toward the axis or midline. The term is most frequently used to describe forces acting on the foot or ankle. Inversion has been equated with adduction in the literature. The term adduction is preferred when describing forces applied to the foot and ankle.
- Abduction: This term indicates motion of a given part away from the midline. Again, terms such as eversion have been used interchangeably with abduction; abduction is preferred when describing forces moving the foot or ankle outward.
- Supination and pronation: Supination and pronation are commonly used for describing the rotation that occurs at the wrist. Technically the foot is pronated when the sole is flat. Pronation can occur to a minimal degree with the forefoot abducted and dorsiflexed. Limited supination is possible. Typically the literature has used the terms pronation and eversion, and supination and inversion, interchangeably. The terms supination and pronation should be reserved for the upper extremity. Eversion and inversion are less confusing when describing foot and ankle position.
- External rotation: The term is typically used to define outward rotation of the foot in relation to the longitudinal axis of the leg. With many athletic injuries the leg actually rotates medially with the foot fixed. Therefore, the foot then is actually rotated in an outward position compared to the leg.

- Varus: Varus indicates rotation, bending, or positioning inward or toward the midline axis. The term should be used to describe position, not motion.
- Valgus: Valgus is used to denote rotation, bending, or positioning away from the axis of the midline. Like varus, the term valgus denotes position.

Soft Tissue Trauma

Injuries affecting the soft tissues of the foot and ankle are common. Cass and Morrey reported and incidence of about 500 ankle sprains per year. Sprains in the foot occur less frequently. Many injuries can be treated conservatively with satisfactory results. Proper imaging evaluation, however, is needed to determine the extent of injury so that chronic instability and function loss can be avoided.

Ankle Ligament Injuries

Certain aspects of ankle anatomy bear repeating, however, to provide a complete discussion of ligamentous trauma.

The distal tibia and fibula are supported in their anatomic relationship by the distal anterior and posterior tibiofibular ligaments and the interosseous membrance Other ligament structures maintain the ankle joint. Medially, the deltiod ligament is triangular and broadens as it extends from the medial malleolus to its talar and calcaneal insertions. The deltoid ligament is composed of an anterior and posterior superficial ligament and an intermediate deep or tibiotalar ligament. The latter ligament is essentially a triangular thickening with a medial capsule. There are three ligaments laterally. The anterior talofibular ligament extends from the anterior fibula to insert in the lateral talus just below the articular surface. With the ankle in a neutral position, this ligament is horizontally oriented and resists internal rotation. Recent studies also indicate that it is significant in resisting varus tilt, particularly with the ankle in plantar flexion. The posterior tibiofibular ligament extends from the posterior fibula to the posterior talus. The clacaneofibular ligament originates at the lateral malleolar tip and inserts on the calcaneus, restricting inversion. The calcaneofibular ligament supports both the ankle and the subtalar joints and is intimately associated with the peroneal tendon sheaths.

Diagnosis of ligament disruption usually requires special studies. Toutine ankle views are not effective in differentiating the types of ankle sprains. Secondary signs, however, are important in determining which additional techniques may be most useful. Patients with grade 1 sprains generally present with mild soft tissue swelling over the lateral malleolus. This can be identified on AP and mortise views. A bright light is frequently needed to evaluate the soft tissues. No fracture or effusion is evident on the lateral view. Grade 2 and 3 sprains have more significant selling that can be identified clinically and on both AP and lateral radiographs. This finding has little value, however. Attempts at correlating ligament injury with the degree of swelling seen radiographically have been unsuccessful. The presence of an effusion in the joint is somewhat useful in that is generally indicates that the capsule is intact. Effusions are best seen on the lateral view. Small avulsion fractures can also be seen on plain films. Measuring the tibiotalar joint to differentiate second- and third-degree sprains is not usually helpful. It the talus is shifted, however, resulting in asymmetry of the ankle mortise, a ligament injury is generally present.

Stress views are less accurate compared to arthrography or tenography. Sauser et al studied 55 patients with stress views and arthrography within 72 hours of injury. They noted that stress views were accurate if talar tilt increased by 10° or more but that the test was only positive in 38% of patients with positive arthrograms.

This decision should be based on clinical findings and whether surgery or treatment modifications will be made as judged from the degree of ligament injury. Surgical intervention is a more important consideration in professional athletes or young active individuals. Generally, assessment of the calcaneofibular ligament is most crucial because conservative treatment is most often used if only the anterior talofibular ligament is torn. Therefore, a stress tenogram is the technique of choice. Computed tomography and MRI are useful in evaluating the tendons around the ankle but, in our experience, are less effective in evaluating the capsule and ligaments.

Ligament injuries also occur in the foot. Gymnastics, long distance running, and aerobic activities are frequently implicated. Inversion injuries, which may mimic typical ankle sprains, may affect the bifurcate ligament, which extends between the calcaneus and cuboid. Other midtarsal ligaments are also stressed in gymnasts and dancers. Diagnosis of these conditions may be difficult clinically.

Cuboid subluxation may be particularly difficult to diagnose. The athlete typically presents with lateral midfoot pain and is unable to run, cut, or jump. Pain or point tenderness may be noted on plantar pressure over the cuboid.

Sinus tarsi syndrome is commonly associated with

inversion injuries of the foot and ankle sprains. The talocalcaneal interosseous ligament carries the hidfoot nerve fibres, and even minor injury may cause significant pain. On physical examination there is point tenderness over the lateral aspect of the sinus tarsi.

Middle-aged joggers commonly develop subluxation of the metatarsophalangeal joint, specifically the second joint. Patients present with metatarsal pain and often have claw toe deformities.

Imaging of ligament injuries of the foot is difficult. Routine radiographs, CT, or conventional tomography may be useful to identify subtle associated avulsion fractures. MRI is useful in specific situations. Diagnostic and therapeutic injections, however, are most useful in localizing the pain and confirming the clinical diagnosis. Fluorscopically monitored injections can be accomplished in all articulations. A mixture of bupivacaine and betamethasone is injected after confirming needle position with a small amount of contrast medium.

Tendon Injuries

Thirteen tendons cross the ankle. These tendons include the peroneus brevis and longus laterally; the Achilles tendon posteriorly; the tibialis posterior, flexor digitorum longus, and flexor hallucis longus medially; and the tibialis anterior, extensor hallucis longus, extensor digitiorum longus, and peroneus tertius anteriorly. All tendons are enclosed in sheaths with the exception of the Achilles tendon. Tendon injury may occur as an isolated event, in association with a fracture, or as a result of previous fracture with degenerative joint disease. Tendons may also rupture in patients on steroid therapy or with chronic inflammatory diseases.

Peroneal Tendons

The peroneal muscles assist in pronation and eversion of the foot. The peroneus brevis tendon is anterior to the peroneus longus as they pass posterior to the lateral malleoulus. In about 80% of patients there is a notch in the fibula that accommodates a portion of the peroneus brevis. In 20% of patients this notch is shallow or absent, which may lead to recurrent subluxation. Thetendons also through the superior and inferior peroneal retinacula. It is between these two structures that they are immediately adjacent to the calcaneofibular ligament. The peroneal tendons share a common sheath to the inferior margin of the superior peroneal retinaculum. At this point the sheath of the peroneus longus separates from that of the peroneus brevis. The peroneus longus progresses inferior to the peroneal tubercle of the calcaneus to the plantar aspect of the foot, where it inserts in the base of the first metatarsal and medial cuneiform. The peroneus brevis passes inferiorly, inserting on the base of the fifth metatarsal. Evaluation of the tendons and normal osseous sulci is easily accomplished with MRI or CT.

Dislocation. Diagnosis of peroneal tendon injury first requires that the problem be considered. Many patients present with a sprained ankle or repeated giving-way, and dislocation of the peroneal tendons is not considered. The mechanism of injury is not clear, but dislocation is probably due to an inversion-dorsiflexion or abduction-dorsiflexion injury. Patients present with pain and swelling over the posterosuperior aspect of the lateral malleolus.

Swelling may make actual palpation of the tendon difficult, and pain with motion can limit the detection of subluxation on physical examination. Routine radiographs will demonstrate soft tissue swelling laterally, but the distribution is not characteristic or different from that of an inversion sprain. A characteristic longitudinal flake fracture along the distal fibular metaphysis is useful when present. This is best seen on the internal oblique view. Murr reported this finding in 15% to 50% of peroneal tendon dislocations. Usually other imaging procedures are more useful. CT, MRI, or tenography should be considered to confirm the diagnosis. CT provides excellent bone detail and is useful in assessing the peroneal notch in the fibula. The tendons are less well demonstrated with CT than with MRI. Subtle tears or complete disruptions are more easily seen on MRI, where the tendons are normally of low signal intensity compared to the high intensity seen in the tendon that has torn. These nonivasive techniques do have disadvantages. For example, if the tendons have returned to normal position or are only slightly displaced, fluoroscopic observation after tenography may be more useful in demonstrating subluxation. This may also be possible to demonstrate with new fast-scan MR techniques.

Rupture of the peroneal tendon. Rupture of the peroneal tendons is not common. The lesion may be overlooked as a cause of ankle instability, however, and therefore the true incidence is not known. Patients may present acutely with an ankle sprain or have symptoms of chronic instability. Cavovarus foot and compartment syndromes have also been reported with peroneal tendon rupture. When the tendons are torn, the patient will be unable effectively to evert the foot.

Routine radiographs are usually not useful. Displacement of the os peroneum, however, may indicate peroneal rupture. Tenography may demonstrate the site of the tear, but because this technique outlines the tendon and does not provide direct assessment it is less useful than MRI. Both CT and MRI have been described as useful techniques for evaluating the peroneal tendons. MRI has superior soft tissue contrast and can define incomplete, complete, and chronic inflammatory changes in both the tendon and the sheath. If a complete tear is present, the tendon ends can be defined as well as the absence of the tendon in its sheath in the torn region. If a partial tear has occurred there will be increased signal intensity in the tendon due to blood and fluid. These findings are most easily demonstrated on T2-weighted or gradient-echo T2* sequences. The contrast of the blood and fluid compared to the normally low-intensity tendon is most striking with these sequences. In patients with old tears the tendon will look thickened with areas of intermediate intensity, and there is often fluid in the tendon sheath. The latter is not seen in normal patients.

Achilles Tendon

The Achilles tendon is the largest and strongest tendon in the foot and ankle. The tendon originates where the gastrocnemius and soleus tendons join and inserts on the posterior calcaneus. In its axial presentation the tendon thickens distally, becoming elliptical with concave anterior and convex posterior surfaces. Approximately 2 to 6 cm above its calcaneal insertion, the fibres in the tendon cross. The posterior fibres course medial to lateral, and the anterior fibres lateral to medial, before inserting in the calcaneus. Most tendon tears occur just above this, perhaps partially because of the reduced blood supply in this region. The Achilles tendon does not have a true tendon sheath.

Acute and chronic inflammation of the Achilles

tendon is common in runners. Up to 11% or runners develop Achilles tendinitis. Inflammation is usually due to errors in training. The injury is also common in request sports and most commonly occurs in 30- to 50-year-old men.

The Achilles tendon, although strong, is commonly torn. Fifty-nine percent of ruptures are related to sports injuries. Ruptures are usually the result of indirect trauma. The injury can occur during athletic activity at any age. It usually occurs in strenuous activities with frequent plantar flexion during raising up on the toes or with pushing off or jumping with the knee extended. Falling or landing on the forefoot, which leads to abrupt dorsiflexion of the foot, can also lead to Achilles rupture. Certain systemic and local conditions predispose to tendon disruption. Gout, systemic lupus erythematosus, rheumatoid arthritis, hyperparathyroidism, chronic renal failure, steroids, and diabetes have all been implicated.

In addition to ruptures, Achilles tendinitis is one of the most common overuse syndromes. Because there is no tendon sheath, the peritenon becomes inflamed. Inflammation is frequently related to footwear and a pronated heel and is seen in runners who use hilly terrain.

Imaging of Achilles tendon pathology can be accomplished with several modalities. Routine radiographs are usually nonspecific. Newmark et al, however, described fracture of a calcaneal osteophyte in association with Achilles tendon avulsion. Low-kilovoltage radiography and Xerox techniques may demonstrate swelling, thickening of the tendon, and irregularity of the pre-Achilles fat or Kager's triangle. These findings are best seen on the lateral view.

Ultrasound can also be effective in elucidating the architecture of the tendon. This requires experience on the part of the examiner and interpreter. Ultrasound images can be difficult to interpret by those who do not routinely use the technique.

CT and MRI, although more expensive than the techniques mentioned above, provide more information about the tendon and surrounding structures. MRI is particularly useful because of its superior soft tissue contrast and ability to image in the axial, sagittal, coronal, and off-axis oblique planes. At the Mayo clinic, we find MRI to be useful in detecting complete, incomplete and old Achilles injuries as well as in evaluating bursitis and other causes of Achilles tendon pathology. The extent of involvement can be assessed accurately with MRI. In addition, patients can be followed to determine whether healing is progressing normally or whether operative intervention is necessary.

Another uncommon problem may mimic and Achilles injury or soft tissue tumour. This situation is created by the presence of an accessory soleus muscle. It is not uncommon for a patients with this anomaly to experience pain after exercise. Either CT or MRI can easily diagnose the condition, but MRI can more easily distinguish the accessory soleus muscle from a soft tissue tumor or hematoma.

Medial Tendons

The posterior tibial, flexor digitorum longus, and flexor hallucis longus tendons make up the medial tendon group and are located anterior to posterior in the above order. The posterior tibial tendon with its tendon sheath passes just posterior to the medial malleolus and lateral to the flexor retinaculum and broadens at its insertion in the navicular tuberosity and base of the medial cuneiform. The flexor digitorum longus takes a similar course proximally, lying between the posterior tibial tendon and the posterior tibial artery. As it turns towards the plantar aspect of the foot, it passes superficially to the flexor hallucis longus before dividing into tendon slips that insert in the bases of the second to fifth distal phalanges. The flexor hallucis longus tendon is located more posteriorly and laterally. It passes through a fibroosseous tunnel beneath the sustentaculum tali and along the medial plantar aspect of the foot to insert in the base of the distal phalanx of the great toe.

Acute rupture of the deltoid ligament is not common. Similarly, the posterior tibial, flexor digitorum longus, and flexor hallucis longus tendons are rarely torn after acute trauma. Zezwart and Davidson have reported posterior tibial tendon rupture in association with bimalleolar fracture.

The posterior tibial tendon is the most commonly injured of the three medial tendons. Injury typically occurs during the pronation phase in running or with rapid changes in direction in basketball, soccer, football, and tennis. Patients present with pain, local tenderness, and swelling, and physical examination may reveal a nonpalpable tendon. Rupture of the posterior tibial tendon can lead to progressive flatfoot deformity, inability to raise up on the toes, and weakness on inversion of the foot.

Routine radiography is usually of little value in patients with medial tendon injuries. Acute traumatic rupture of the posterior tibial tendon has been described in association with medial malleolar fractures. The fracture is a mirror image of the flake fracture seen with peroneal tendon dislocation. It occurs longitudinally along the distal medial tibial metaphysis. Posterior tibial tendon rupture may present with an increased tolocalcaneal angle on the AP and lateral view. These findings, along with soft tissue swelling, are the only plain film findings that might suggest the diagnosis. In patients with chronic disease and inflammation, the stress tenogram may show changes in the posterior tibial or adjacent tendon sheaths. The structure of the tendon is better demonstrated with CT or MRI, however. In our experience MRI has been most useful in assessing the nature and degree of posterior tibial tendon pathology.

Rupture of the flexor digitorum and flexor hallucis longus tendons occurs less frequently but can present with similar clinical findings. Garth reported rupture of the flexor hallucis longus in ballet dancers and soccer players. Patients presented with swelling, tenderness, and crepitation near the sustentaculum tali. Symptoms were increased with flexion and extension of the great toe.

Tenography of the flexor hallucis longus is tedious because of the difficulty in localizing the tendon with the needle tip. Therefore, MRI or CI is more useful.

Anterior Tendons

Anteriorly the anterior tibial, extensor hallucis longus, and extensor digitorum longus tendons are all enclosed in tendon sheaths. Acute tears are unusual, but in patients with previous fractures, degenerative arthritis, or other predisposing factors tendon rupture can occur, Chronic inflammation or more significant involvement of the anterior tibial tendon is not uncommon in runners. Rupture of the anterior tibial tendon usually occurs as it exits the superior retinaculum. The distal segment retracts and can be palpated between the superior and inferior retinacula.

Clinically there is pain and swelling over the ankle anteriorly. There may also be decreased dorsiflextion of the foot on physical examination.

Radiographically patients will demonstrate minimal to prominent soft tissue swelling anteriorly. This is most easily identified on the lateral and oblique views.

Hindfoot Pain

Hindfoot and/or heel pain is common in athletes. For purposes of discussion, it is useful to consider four different areas plantar, posterior, lateral, and medial.

Plantar Pain

The most common problem resulting in plantar pain is fasciitis. The condition is noted in 7% of runners. In the acute phase there is more focal pain at the medial calcaneal attachment, but with prolonged symptoms the pain and area of tenderness on physical examination become more diffuse. The condition is more common with cavus foot or excessive pronation.

Routine radiography may demonstrate distortion of soft tissue planes or periostitis. These changes are most easily appreciated on the lateral view. Although radionuclide scans may be useful, MRI is most effective for differentiation of inflammation from ruptures of the plantar fascia.

Medial calcaneal nerve entrapment may also lead to plantar pain. The condition is most often noted in runners, and some investigators postulate the syndrome is caused by inflammation of the nerve as it passes through the abductor hallucis. MRI is the most useful modality for evaluating plantar pain. Coronal and sagittal T2-weighted images are most effective.

Posterior Pain

Posterior heel pain may be related to Achilles tendon injury or inflammation or bursitis. The first two were discussed previously. Retrocalcaneal burisitis is an inflammation of the bursa located between the Achilles and posterosuperior calcaneus. Patients with increased calcaneal inclination or cavus foot are more likely to be affected.

Lateral Pain

Lateral heel pain occurs infrequently. Peroneal tendon injury, described above, and sural nerve entrapment should be considered in this setting. Nerve entrapment may be caused by tendon sheath ganglia or avulsion fractures that cause entrapment of the nerve, which runs posterior to the peroneal tendons. MRI in the axial and sagittal planes is most useful for imaging this region.

Medial Pain

Medial tendon injuries were described previously. Tarsal tunnel syndrome is caused by irritation of the tibial nerve as it passes beneath the flexor retinaculum. Chronic trauma due to recurrent sprains and fractures or fracture dislocations may lead to tarsal tunnel syndrome.

Patients typically present with burning pain medially or heelparesthesia. Symptoms increase with weight bearing. MRI is most useful for evaluation of this and other medial hindfoot syndromes. Axial and sagittal T2-weighted images are most useful in this regard.

Forefoot Pain

Forefoot pain is a common problem in athletes. Those conditions responsible for these symptoms, excluding fractures, are reviewed below.

- Metatarsalgia: Metatarsal pain may be due to a long second metatarsal and a hypermobile first metatarsal. This localized form of forefoot pain usually correlates with a metatarsal pad insert. More generalized metatarsal pain is evident in athletes with a tight Achilles tendon or anterior ankle impingement. Surgical correction may be required in the latter.
- Sesamoiditis: Sesamoid pain syndromes are common in runners. The mdeial and lateral hallucis brevis. Their function is to elevate the first metatarsal head to disperse impact forces, to protect the flexor hallucis tendon, and to increase the mechanical advantage of the flexor hallucis brevis tendon. The sesamoids may become inflamed or fractured or may undergo osteonecrosis. Patients with simple sesamioiditis usually respond to rest and longitudinal arch support. For those who do not respond, more significant injury must be excluded.
- Osteochondritis: Forefoot pain in athletes may also be due to osteonecrosis of the metatarsal head. The second metatarsal head is most commonly involved. Women are affected more frequently than men.
- Metatarsophalangeal subluxation and synovitis: Synovitis and/or subluxation of the metatarsophalangeal joints results in local tenderness, swelling, and pain with passive flexion. Synovitis is common in football players, especially those playing on artificial surfaces. The second metatarsophalangeal joint is most commonly affected; it is followed in frequency by the first and third joints. If the condition persists, hammertoe or medial or lateral translocation may develop. Subluxation more often occurs in middle-aged

male joggers; the second metatarsal is most commonly involved. Other forefoot pain syndromes, neuromas, and stress fractures must be excluded.

- Hallux rigidus: Athletes frequently develop hallux rigidus, usually as a result of chronic trauma. Symptoms usually occur with starting from a squatting stance, such as in football or track. Hard-soled shoes may be helpful. In certain cases surgical correction may be indicated.
- Neuromas: Neuromas are due to chronic trauma to the interdigital nerve. Symptoms are commonly noted between the third and fourth metatarsal heads. Paresthesia and numbness is the sensory distribution of the nerve are common. On examination, pain is elicited by placing pressure on the plantar aspect of the foot while compressing the metatarsal heads. Generally, properly fitting footwear or direct injection with anaesthetic and steroid will be successful. Surgery may be required in certain cases, however. In this setting, imaging is useful before consideration and planning of surgery.

Imaging of forefoot problems should begin with radiographs in the oblique and standing AP and lateral projections. Normal angles, joint congruency, and phalangeal deformities provide valuable clues to injury or foot deformities such as cavus foot that predispose to certain pain syndromes. The position and appearance of the sesamoids should be carefully assessed. Sesamoid are useful in patients with suspected abnormalities.

When routine radiographs are normal, radionuclide scans are useful to define early injuries such as stress fractures, sesamoiditis, or early osteonecrosis. Findings on bone scan can allow more specific imaging with CT or tomoraphy to define the lesion more effectively. Recently, MRI has become a frequent second choice after routine films. MRI can clearly define soft tissue lesions such as neuromas as well as osseous abnormalities.

Ankle Fractures

Management of foot and ankle fractures is a common problem for orthopaedic surgeons, emergency department physicians, family practice physicians, and radiologists. Imaging plays an important role in assessing the degree of bone and soft tissue injury and in following the healing process.

The detection of most fractures is not difficult. Detection of subtle fractures and evaluation of the extent of soft tissue injury, however, may be more difficult. Thus it is essential for those interpreting images to be aware of the manner in which various fractures and soft tissue injuries present so that the images can be evaluated correctly and thoroughly. Soft tissue changes may be the only clue to a subtle fracture of ligament rupture. Soft tissue swelling, obliteration of the fat planes or the pre-Achilles fat triangle, and the presence of an effusion can be useful in identifying the location of subtle fractures.

It is also important to understand the clinical significance of certain fracture patterns. Fractures may be complete or incomplete. The latter are more common in children. Avulsion fractures occur at the insertion of ligaments or tendons.

Pediatric Ankle Fractures

Ankle fractures may be simple or complex with associated ligament rupture. The latter are more common in adults. Generally, fractures in patients older than 15 to 16 years of age are classified and treated on the basis of adult criteria.

The appearance of ankle fractures in children depends upon the age, relationship of the ligaments to the epiphytes, and mechanisms of injury. Distal diaphyseal and metaphyseal fractures are frequently incomplete. In most cases there is a posterior cortical break with buckling of the anterior cortex above the growth plate. Fractures of the distal tibia and fibula frequently involve the growth plates. The distal tibia epiphysis is the second most common site for growth plate fracture. In Rogers' series, 25% of 118 physeal injuries involved the distal tibia or fibula. Physeal fractures can result in growth or articular deformity if proper diagnosis and treatment are not implemented.

There are two types of epiphyses. Pressure epiphyses are located in the ends of long bones and are subject to weight-bearing forces and forces acting on the joint. Traction epiphyses occur at sites of muscle or tendon insertions. The latter are not directly associated with weight bearing. The pressure epiphyses of the distal tibia and fibula contribute 45% and 40%, respectively, of the growth of the tibia and fibula. The proximal epiphyses of the tibia contribute 55%, and those of the proximal fibula contribute 60%. The distal tibial and fibular epiphyses appear at age 2. The tibial epiphysis fuses by age 15 in girls and 17 in boys. The fibular epiphysis remains open longer and fuses at age 20.

Histologically the growth plate is divided into four zones. Progressing distally from the metaphysis, these zones include the zone of provisional calcification, the hypertrophic cartilage zone, the proliferating zone, and the resting zone. The cartilage cells are surrounded by longitudinally oriented collagen fibres and a chondrotin sulfate matrix. This substance is less abundant in the hypertrophic zone, which at least partially explains why this zone is the most susceptible to fracture. The blood supply to the epiphysis and metaphysis of the long bones is separate, with the exception of the proximal readial and femoral epiphyses. Therefore, when fracture of the growth plate occurs the blood supply is generally not disrupted. This spares the proliferating zone, and normal growth can occur after healing.

The same forces the cause fracture and/or ligament disruption in adults also cause fractures in children. In children the growth plates are two to five times weaker than the ligaments, so that fractures of the physes occur more commonly than ligament injuries. The fracture patterns that evolve are thus related to age, the ligamentous attachments, and the type of force applied. Growth plate fractures are more common during the first year and the rapid growth phases in the early teens.

The most commonly used classification system for physical injuries was described by Salter and Harris. This classification is useful because of its prognostic significance and easy-to-use radiographic patterns. Type I fractures are due to separation of the epiphysis with the fracture line confined to the growth plate. The fracture usually extends through the hypertrophic zone and does not involve the epiphysis or metaphysis. In Rogers' of injury may be subtle radiographically. Comparison radiographs of the uninjured ankle may be helpful. Type I injuries are uncommon in athletes and tend to occur more commonly in children younger than 5 years of age. The prognosis is generally excellent.

Type II fractures are the most common. This fracture extends through the growth plate for a variable distance before exiting through the metaphysis. Type II fractures occur more commonly in patients older than 10 years of age. Eversion or inversion injuries with forced abduction or adduction of the foot have been implicated in this ankle fracture.

Type III fractures are intraarticular, extending through the epiphysis and entering the growth plate, where they exit through the hypertrophic zone. The metaphysis is spared. This injury is usually due to an intraarticular shearing force.

Type IV fractures extend from the articular surface of the epiphysis through the growth plate and exit through the metaphysis. Complete reduction of this fracture is essential to prevent growth disturbances. This fracture makes up 10% of Salter-Harris fractures.

Type V fractures are the result of compression injuries that cause impaction of the growth plate. The ankle and knee are commonly involved. The prognosis is guarded with type V fractures. These fractures are uncommon.

Other classifications have also been applied to growth plate fractures. Crenshaw proposed a classification similar to that of Salter and Harris that is frequently used because of its simplicity. Injuries are categorized according to forces applied: external rotation, abduction, adduction, plantar flexion, and direct trauma. With this approach the pattern of injury can be used in fracture reduction. Fractures are reduced by gently reversing the direction of the mechanism of injury noted radiographically.

External rotation injuries occur when the foot is subjected to external rotation forces. This tress leads to fracture of the posterolateral tibial physis and often a fracture of the fibula above the growth plate. Abduction injuries result in Salter-Harris I or II fractures of the anterolateral tibia. The direction of stress and talar shift usually displaces the fragment laterally. Talar forces may lead to associated fibular fractures. Adduction forces are similar to inversion injuries, placing tension on the lateral ligament complex. This results in avulsion or distal fibular physical fractures. The force, if continued, will cause impaction of the talus against the medial malleolus, leading to a Salter-Harris III or IV fracture of the medial malleolus. Plantar flexion injuries lead to posterior epiphyseal injuries. By definition there is no external rotation force, and therefore no associated fibular fracture is evident. The Crenshaw fracture patterns are most common during the 12th year, and there is a significantly higher incidence in boys.

More recently, the Lauge-Hansen system has been combined with the Salter-Harris system. The former is an accurate method commonly applied to adult ankle injuries and is discussed later. Dias and Tachdjian studied 71 patients with their combined classification system, and only 4 patients did not properly fit the categories. This classification, like the Lauge-Hansen system, is based on the position of the foot during the injury and the direction of the abnormal force.

Several ankle fractures do not fit into this classification. A Salter-Harris III of the distal tibia is usually due to external rotation forces. This fracture is generally seen in the lateral portion of the tibia. Triplane is generally seen in the lateral portion of the tibia. Triplanc fractures do not fit the original Dias-Tachdjian classification. The injury is believed to be due to external rotation with or without associated plantar flexion. The fracture consists of three fragments instead of the two fragments seen with most growth plate fractures. The first fragment involves the anterolateral portion of the tibial epiphysis and looks like a Salter-Harris III injury. The second fragment is the remainder of the tibial epiphysis with the metaphyseal attachment. The third fragment is the tibial metaphysis. The fracture has a characteristic radiographic appearance. On the AP view it has the appearance. On the AP view it has the appearance of a Salter-Harris III fracture, and on the lateral view it resembles a Salter-Harris II fracture of the distal tibia. The incidence of triplane fractures is not high. Cooperman et al noted an incidence of 6% in a series of 237 patients with epiphyseal fractures of the ankle. In reality the fracture behaves like a Salter-Harris IV, and since its original description many investigators hold that it is often only a two-part fracture. The medial malleolus and anteromedial portion of the epiphysis remain attached to the tibial metaphysis and form one fragment. The second fragment is the lateral portion of the epiphysis with the lateral metaphysical attachment. Other variations of he triplance fracture have also been described.

The so-called juvenile Tillaux fracture is a Salter-Harris III fracture of the distal lateral tibia. The fragment is displaced by the distal tibiofibular ligaments when the foot is externally rotated.

Most epiphysical injuries can be clearly defined on the routine ankle trauma series: AP, lateral, and morise views. In most cases the entire tibia and fibula should be included on the films so that a high fibular fracture is not overlooked. Fractures of the fibular physis, the most common ankle fracture, may be very subtle. Usually Salter-Harris I or, more commonly, II fractures are best seen on the mortise view. When the foot is internally rotated 15° to 20°, the fibula is viewed clear of the tibia. This fracture, however, should be suspected in any child with swelling and point tenderness over the growth plate. When no other fractures are evident the patient can be splinted, and a repeat study in 10 to 14 days will often demonstrate the fracture line more clearly. Slight perosteal callus may also be evident at this time. When a Salter-Harris III or IV fracture is present medially, one should assume that the growth plate or the lateral ligaments are damaged or that an avulsion fracture may be present. Salter-Harris I and II fractures of the distal tibia may also present with subtle radiographic findings. Comparison views on an approach similar to the one described above can be used to evaluate these fractures.

More complex physical injuries, especially triplane fractures or comminuted epiphyseal fractures, can be better evaluated with CT or MRI. These techniques clearly demonstrate the epiphyseal fragmentation and distal tibiofibular relationships. As is the case for adults, it is important to define the degree of articular involvement, note any articular irregularity, and clearly define the degree of separation of the fracture fragments. Displacement of more than 2 mm has significant treatment implications.

Adult Ankle Fractures

Complete evaluation of ankle fractures in adults includes assessment of the fracture fragments and accurate description of associated ligament injuries. Evaluation of bone and soft tissue involvement is important in determining the mechanism of injury, which in turn has significant treatment implications.

When evaluating ankle fractures it is common to consider the bones and ligaments a ring-like structure in the coronal plane. The ring is made up of the medial malleolus, tibial plafond, distal tibiofibular ligaments and syndemosis, lateral malleolus, lateral ligaments, talus, and medial ligaments. Breaks in the ring commonly occur at five sites either alone or in combination. Shift of the talus indicates disruption of the ring at more than one site. The five common sites of injury include the lateral malleolus, lateral ligaments, deltoid ligaments, medial malleolus, and syndesmosis. Fractures of the tibial plafond occur after axial loading with various degrees of plantar flexion.

Clinical Features

After ankle injury, patients generally present with various degrees of pain, swelling, and ecchymosis depending to some degree on the significance of the injury. The incidence of swelling and presence of ecchymosis is somewhat higher when fractures are present, but this is not a reliable clinical finding. With incomplete injuries and stable fractures weight bearing is usually still possible. Weight bearing is more difficult or impossible with unstable fractures.

Most ankle fractures occur as a result of inversion or eversion forces. The mechanism of injury is rarely pure, however. Most often abduction, adduction, lateral rotation, of axial loading occur in addition to eversion or inversion.

The value of classifications for ankle fractures is that they have a significant impact on treatment, prognosis, and establishing the mechanism of injury. Classifications must also be workable and easy to remember. With this in mind, various classifications have been developed for ankle fractures. The more commonly employed classifications are those proposed by Lauge-Hansen and Weber. The former is accurate in predicting the mechanism of injury and extent of ligament involvement. Therefore, it is recommended to radiologists so that the description of the injury can be most accurate. The Weber classification is not as complex but is frequently used because of its value in planning appropriate therapy.

The Lauge-Hansen classification was devised with the use of cadaver specimens. It is based on the position of the foot at the time of injury and the direction of the injuring force. With this system, four basic categorise of injury are described. The classification considers different levels of injury in each category on the basis of the degree of the force and the length of time for which it is applied.

Supination-adduction injuries cause traction on the lateral ligaments, resulting in either a ligament tear of an avulsion fracture of the lateral malleolus. The fracture is generally transverse and below the joint level. If the force is sufficient, the talus can impact against the medial malleolus. If an oblique fracture of the medial malleolus is evident but not fracture is seen in the lateral malleolus, one can assume that the lateral ligaments are disrupted.

PREVENTIVE MEASURES

1. Wear the correct shoes for your particular activity.

2. Wear hiking shoes or boots in rough terrain.

3. Don't continue to wear any sports shoe if it is worn unevenly.

4. The toe box in "steel-toe" shoes should be deep enough to accommodate your toes comfortably.

5. Always wear hard-top shoes when operating a lawn mower or other grass-cutting equipment.

6. Don't walk barefoot on paved streets or sidewalks.

7. Watch out for slippery floors at home and at work. Clean up obviously dangerous spills immediately.

8. If you get up during the night, turn on a light. Many fractured toes and other foot injuries occur while attempting to find one's way in the dark.

HOW TO CARE FOR YOUR ANKLE SPRAIN

What is an ankle sprain?

The injury that occurs when your foot "rolls," or turns in on itself, is called an ankle sprain. In this injury, the ligaments that hold the ankle and foot bones in place are stretched and weakened.

What should be done after an ankle sprain?

Many doctors recommend that you use the RICE treatment after a sprain:

R= Rest. Stay off the injured ankle to help it heal. This also helps prevent further injury. Your doctor might have you use crutches if walking is too painful. Stay off

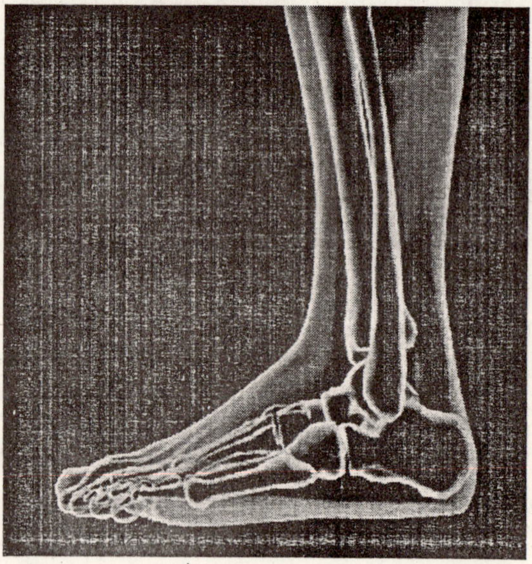

your feet most of the time until you can walk without pain.

I = Ice. Ice helps keep the swelling down. It also helps to reduce pain. Put an ice pack on the ankle for 15 minutes. Take the ice off for 10 minutes. Put ice back on for 10 minutes. Then use ice for 15 minutes at a time three times a day for two more days.

C= Compression. Compression (wrapping the ankle with a strip of elastic cloth) will help decrease swelling and support your ankle. You can use an elastic wrap from the drugstore, or get an air splint from your doctor. (Your doctor will show you how to use it.) Be careful not to wrap the ankle too tightly. That would slow the blood flow to your foot. Use the elastic bandage for 1 to 2 days.

E = Elevation. Keeping your foot raised helps decrease pain and swelling. When you elevate your ankle, try to keep it around the level of your heart. Lying on a couch with pillows under your foot is better than sitting in a chair with your foot on a footstool. Try to keep your foot elevated for 2 to 3 hours a day.

What should be taken for pain?

Most doctors recommend anti-inflammatory medicines such as ibuprofen (brand names: Advil, Medipren, Motrin, Nuprin), naprosyn (brand name: Aleve) or ketoprofen (brand name: Orudis KT). You can also take acetaminophen (brand names: Tylenol, Datril, Panadol), although this medicine isn't an anti-inflammatory.

After my ankle sprain heals, what can I do to strengthen my ankle?

It's important for you to strengthen your ankle after a sprain. This helps prevent another injury. Use elastic tubing (available at drug stores and most sports equipment stores) and follow a few basic exercises, described below. Do 10 repetitions of each exercise (this is called a "set"); do three sets of each exercise, twice a day. For example, in the morning, you'll do 40 repetitions (four exercises, 10 times each) three times. In the evening, you'll do another 40 repetitions three times.

EXERCISES AFTER AN ANKLE SPRAIN

Sit on a firm chair, or stand up. Loop one end of the tubing around the ball of the foot with the injured ankle. Hold the other end of the tubing in your hand. Put your heel on the floor. Stretch the tubing by pushing down with your foot, the way you push on the gas pedal of a car.

Sit on a firm chair, or stand up. Loop one end of the tubing around the leg of a sturdy table. Loop the other end of the tubing around the foot with the injured ankle. Stretch the tubing by pulling up with your foot (lifting up your foot), using your ankle, as if you were trying to pull the table toward you. (This motion is the opposite of trying to "step on the gas.")

Sit on a firm chair, or stand up. Loop one end of the tubing around the leg of a sturdy table. Loop the other end of the tubing around the foot with the injured ankle. Stretch the tubing by moving your foot out to the side, away from the leg of the table.

Sit on a firm chair, or stand up. Loop one end of the tube around the leg of a sturdy table. Loop the other end of the tubing around the foot with the injured ankle. Stretch the tubing by moving your foot in to the middle, toward your good ankle.

You can also do these exercises with your uninjured ankle, to keep it strong and less likely to sprain.

10

Spine Injuries

The human spine is a remarkable structure. During athletic activity the spine is able to withstand tremendous stresses and forces and at the same time remain quite flexible and mobile. The spine, or vertebral column, encases and provides protection for the spinal cord. Trauma to the spine can produce devastating athletic injuries.

These injuries can be fatal or can cause irreversible damage to the spinal cord, resulting in permanent paralysis. To accurately assess and care for injuries to this area of the body, it is imperative that the athletic trainer possess a thorough understanding of the anatomic and mechanical characteristics of the spine.

ANATOMY OF THE SPINE

The spine consists of 33 vertebrae, which are subdivided into seven cervical, twelve thoracic, five lumbar, five sacral, and four coccygeal vertebrae. The 24 nonfused vertebrae lying superior to the scrum increase in size from the first cervical through the fifth lumbar. Between each of these vertebrae is an intervertebral disc. Discs act as shock absorbers and allow movement between adjacent vertebrae.

Inrtervertebral discs

Each intervertebral disc consists of two structures,

the tough outer annulus fibrosus and the semisolid central nucleus purposes. The annulus fibrosus connects the bodies of adjacent vertebrae through obliquely arranged layers fibrocartilage. Each layer of fibres is perpendicular to the adjacent layers.

This arrangement gives the disc strength and elasticity. The annulus fibrosus is thicker anteriorly and laterally. This fact explains the larger number of posterior disc herniation. The nucleus pulposus is a gelatinous substance located in the centre of the disc. It has a strong capacity to retain water.

Muscles acting on the vertebral column

The vertebral column, in part or as a whole, may be moved or acted upon by numerous muscles or muscle groups. Some muscles have both their origin and insertion on the spine and act directly on the column, whereas others act only indirectly on the spine and have

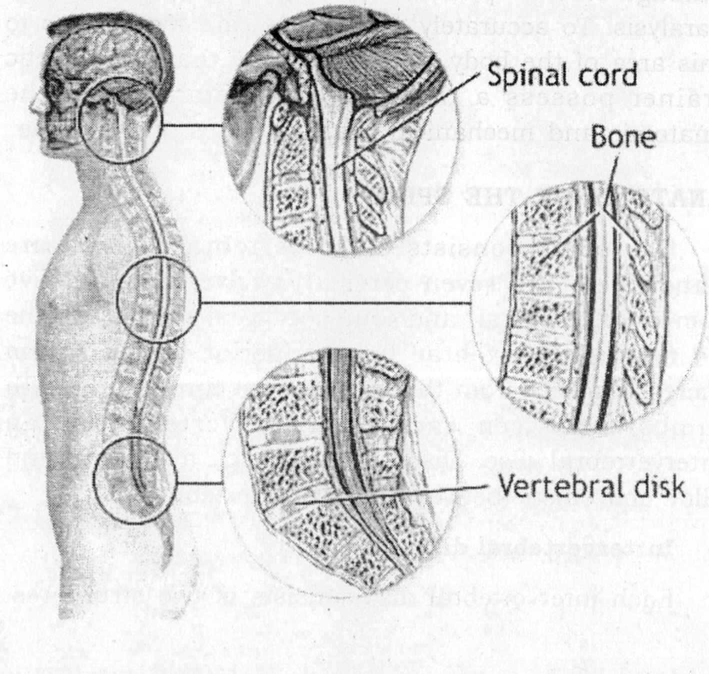

their origin or insertion on some other bone or soft tissue component. The superficial muscles of the back are, as a group, related to the upper limbs.

The complex deep, or intrinsic, muscles of the back extend from the base of the skull to the pelvis on each side of the body. They control the movements of the vertebral column. The short intrinsic muscles tend to steady adjoining vertebrae during movements of the column as a whole. The long intrinsic muscles or muscle groups are more involved in gross movements of the entire spine.

Dermatomes

Each spinal nerve supplies sensory fibres to areas of skin on the body surface that are arranged in a definite segmental pattern. Each strip of skin supplied by a given spinal nerve is called a dermatome. Although there is considerable overlap in the innervation of each dermatome, sensation in each band is associated with a particular spinal nerve; loss of sensation in a dermatome segment suggests injury to the spinal nerve supplying that segment.

If, for example, there is a loss of skin sensation in a band that circle the trunk at the level of the umbilicus, a physician would assume injury to the spinal nerve root supplying that area. Each segment of the spine is discussed separately in more detail along with the athletic injuries common to each area. Type and severity of athletic injuries varies, depending on which segment of the spine is involved. As a result, the evaluation and subsequent management must be specific to the area injured.

Ligaments of the vertebral column

The bodies of adjacent vertebrae are connected by

strong ligaments. Two important longitudinal ligaments can be identified through the entire length of the spinal column. The anterior longitudinal ligament is a strong, band like structure composed of several layers of fibres that extends along and is firmly attached to the anterior surface of each vertebral body.

It extends from the base of the skull to the scrum. The posterior longitudinal ligament lies on the inside of the vertebral canal on the posterior surface of the bodies of the vertebrae. It is principally a structure that serves to connect the intervertebral discs.

It consists of smooth, glistening fibres that commence on the body of the axis and continue downward to the sacrum. In addition, the ligamenta flava bind the laminae of adjacent vertebrae firmly together. Spinous processes are connected by interspinous ligaments.

The transverse processes of adjacent vertebrae are connected by the specialized ligamentum nuchae, which extends downward from the external occipital protuberance at the base of the skull to join the spinous processes of all seven cervical vertebrae.

This strong and important fan-shaped ligament lies in the midline and forms a septum between the neck muscles. The extension of this ligament, the supraspinous ligament, connects the tips of the rest of the vertebrae down to the sacrum.

Spinal cord

The spinal cord is a continuation of the motor and sensory pathways from the brain to the body and extremities. It is encased and protected within the bony spinal canal. The spinal cord is surrounded by the meninges, cerebrospinal fluid, a cushion of adipose tissue, and blood vessels.

The cord extends from the foreman magnum to the lower border of the first lumbar vertebra, an average distance of 17 to 18 inches in the adult. Although the spinal cord terminates at the level of the first lumbar vertebrae, lumbar, sacral, and coccygeal nerve roots continue to descend in the canal. This gives the lower end of the spinal cord, with its attached spinal nerve roots, the appearance of a horse's tail, and prompted early anatomists to describe it as the cauda equina.

The spinal cord is oval and less than ½ inch in diameter. It tapers slightly from above downward and is extremely sensitive to injury. For example, it is said that if you were to drop a quarter on an exposed spinal cord from a height of 12 inches neural function distal to the point of impact would be severely impaired. There are 31 pairs of spinal nerves connected to the spinal cord.

Cervical spine

The cervical spine is of paramount importance to the athletic trainer. This area of the spine has greater flexibility than any other vertebral segment. There are seven cervical vertebrae by the presence of a foreman through their by the presence of a foreman through their transverse processes. With the exception of the first cervical vertebrae, or atlas, each component of the cervical spine is characterized by the following component parts:

1. Two transverse processes, which project laterally from each vertebra.

2. A central opening called the verterbal foreman, formed by the junction of the lamina with the body. This is the opening through which the spinal cord passes.

3. The body, which is a flat mass located anteriorly

and centrally. In the cervical vertebrae the body tends to be wider from side to side than in the anteroposterior diameter.

4. The spinous process, a sharp palpable process that projects posteriorly and inferiorly from each vertebra.

5. Inferior articular facets, which are directed anteriorly and inferiorly.

6. Two lamina, which join the spinous process on either side with the body.

7. Superior articular facets, which are directed superiorly and posteriorly.

The bodies of adjacent vertebrae articulate with each other through the intervention of the intervertebral discs and through their articular facets or processes. The upper and lower pairs of articular processes between vertebrated are arranged vertically, except in the cervical spine.

In the cervical spine the more transverse arrangement of the articular facets between adjacent vertebrae makes dislocation possible without fracture. It is not possible for a simple dislocation to occur elsewhere in the spinal column because of the vertical direction of the articular processes.

With the exception of the cervical spine, any dislocation injury must be a fracture dislocation, because the articular processes must break before the vertebral bodies can be separated. The atlas has large oval and concave facets that articular with the occipital condyles of the skull.

Nodding and lateral flexion movements occur at the atlanto-occipital joint. The axis is characterized by the dens on the superior aspect of its body. Rotation of the skull occurs at the atlanto-axial joint, with the dens acting as a pivot. In addition to the longitudinal ligaments and articular capsules, a number of specialized ligaments help to stabilize the articulations between the skull and atlas and between the atlas and axis.

The transverse ligament of the atlas, for example, protects the spinal cord in certain types of cervical fracture by limiting backward displacement of the dens into the vertebral canal. Rotation of the skull is limited by the lateral odontoid or "check" ligaments. These very strong fibrous bands extend from each occipital condyle at the base of the skull to the dens, or odontoid process, of the axis.

Cervical spine injuries

Injuries to the cervical spine can be the most serious of athletic injuries. These injuries range in severity from minor neck pain to complete paralysis or death. It is imperative that the athletic trainer protect the athlete from further injury whenever an injury to the cervical spine is suspected.

Ill-advised assessment procedures and improper handling and transporting manoeuvres may cause irreparable spinal cord damage to an athlete who has suffered a cervical spine fracture or dislocation. Therefore utmost caution must be used in evaluating, treating and handling the athlete who has suffered an injury to the neck region.

This is one of the body with which it is certainly better to be conservative and cautious in your assessment of injury rather than to risk a lifetime of paralysis, or possibly death, for the athlete. Injuries to the cervical spine can involve the vertebrae, intervertebral discs, ligaments, muscles, nerve roots, or spinal cord.

These structures can be injured by various mechanisms. The most common mechanism of injury to the neck is forced movements of the head on the cervical spine. This can occur when the athlete receives a blow to the head that forces the neck beyond its normal limits of motion, resulting in forced hyperextension, flexion, lateral flexion, rotation, or a combination of these movements.

The contractile tissue surrounding the cervical spine may be stretched or strained while attempting to resist this forced movement. If forced movement is severe or violent enough, serious injuries to the neck, such as fractures of dislocations, may occur. Injuries to the cervical spine may also be the result of cervical compression.

When an athlete receives a head-on blow, the force is transmitted through the cervical spine and may cause vertebral fracture or dislocation. The neck can also be injured by a direct blow. This mechanism usually results in contusions or bruising about the neck but can result in a serious spinal cord injury if the blow is violent enough.

The most common injuries to the neck are sprains and strains, which often occur simultaneously. These injuries vary in severity. Slight trauma may result in very mild injuries of little consequence. In these cases, the athlete will express no feelings of weakness or instability. Although there may be tenderness and pain at the site of the injury, the athlete can easily demonstrate a normal range of motion in the neck.

In more severe injuries, the athlete will usually resist moving the neck through a full range of motion.

With the more severe injuries there will be localized pain and muscle spasm, and the athlete may complain of an insecure feeling about the neck. Injuries resulting in moderate to severe neck sprains and strains should be referred to a physician for further evaluation.

Thoracic spine

The basic anatomic characteristics typical of vertebrae in general are easily identified in the 12 components of the thoracic spine. The thoracic vertebrae show the least modification of the basic patter. Transitional changes in appearance occur in an individual vertebra toward the cervical and lumbarends of the thoracic region.

The first and twelfth thoracic vertebrae are distinctly transitional. Whereas T1 has a long and almost horizontal spinous process, the spine on T12 is short and broadened. The remaining spinous processes of thoracic verterabe are long and tend to slope sharply downward. The heart-shaped of a typical thoracic vertebra is intermediate in size between those of the cervical and lumbar segments.

Unique costal facets are found on each side of thoracic vertebrae at the junction of the body and lamina. Adjacent facets of contiguous vertebrae from an articular socket for the head of a rib. These facets are found only on thoracic vertebrae. The thoracic spine is the most stable section of the vertebral column.

Although a considerable range of motion is possible, including flexion, extension, rotation, and lateral bending movements, and actual displacement between vertebrae is limited. Stability of the thoracic spine results from the obliquently set articular facets, the thin intervertebral discs, the overlapping of the long spinous processes, and the attachment of the ribs.

In addition, the well-developed anterior longitudinal and posterior longitudinal ligaments effectively limit motion. The functional price paid for stability in this region is restricted motion between individual vertebrae.

Thoracic spine injuries

The most common athletic injuries to the thoracic spine are contusions, sprains, and strains. Contusions caused by a blow to the thoracic area more commonly involve the parapsinal muscles, those muscles lateral to the spinous processes. Sprains and strains may be caused by overstretching of the soft tissue surrounding the thoracic vertebrae or by violent muscular contraction against resistance.

On examination it may be difficult to distinguish between a sprain or strain. Witl. either of these injuries there may be tenderness, spasm, and increased pain on active contraction or stretching. An, athlete with a moderate to severe injury may exhibit a very stiff back and may resist any motion or movement of the thoracic spine.

Serious injuries to the thoracic spine are extremely rare in athletic activity. Fractures or dislocations are unusual because of the stable anatomy previously described. The most common serious injury is a compression fracture to the body of one of the thoracic vertebrae.

The mechanism of injury is usually forced forward flexion of the thoracic spine, which compresses the anterior portion spine, which compresses the anterior portion of adjacent vertebral bodies. Typically, the athlete will give a history of sharp forward flexion, resulting in a jackknifing effect. This can occur as an athlete falls violently on the buttocks or is forced into extreme flexion of the thoracic spine.

An athlete with a compression fracture will usually have no neurologic complaints and will be able to move around and even walk. However, the athlete will complain of constant localized pain, which may be increased with any movement of this area of the spine. The athlete should be referred for further evaluation and radiographs.

Lumbar spine

The five lumbar vertebrae differ from the thoracic vertebrae in their larger size and absence of costal facets. The massive bodies of these vertebrae are designed to stabilize and accommodate the increasing body weight that must be supported the increasing body weight that must be supported toward the lower end of the spinal column.

The prominent lumbar curve, an anterior convexity somewhat deeper in women than men, helps to project the weight of the torso onto the lower limbs. Progressive changes in appearance of specific verterbral components through of the bodies from side to side and a marked separation between articular processes.

The articular processes of lumbar vertebrae are oriented to facilitate a considerable range of movement, particularly in flexion, extension, and side-to-side bending. They do not, however, permit axial rotation.

Lumbosacral joint

The body weight is supported by the opposing surfaces of the first sacral and fifth lumbar vertebra and by the two articulations between the superior sacral and inferior lumbar articular processes. Articulations between the last, or fifth lumbar vertebra and the sacrum are similar to the joints that exists between the movable vertebrae in the spine above.

However, the intervertebral disc located between L5 and the sacrum is very thick, especially along its anterior border. This articulation is the meeting place of the movable lumbar spine above with the fixed and rigid sacrum below. It is notorious as a frequent site of pain.

The lumbosacral angle has a rather extensive normal range of variation but averages about 120° in most adults. The anterior surface of the lumbosacral joint lies in a straight line directly below the occipital condyles when the body is erect and the posture normal.

The joint also marks the termination of the lumbar convexity and the commencement of the sacral concavity. The fifth lumbar vertebra may be joined in whole or in part to the sacrum. This is known as sacralization of the fifth lumbar vertebra. The condition is often devoid of symptoms but may be the cause of back pain in some athletes. The two bones entering into the lumbosacral articulation are held together by a host of very strong ligaments.

Sprains are common, however if this body areas is subjected to direct blows or sudden twisting movements. Lordosis increases the possibility of ligament sprains in this area. The major ligaments associated with the lumbosacral junction can be evaluated by asking the athlete to lie supine on a table and hyperflex both thighs on the abdomen. This position will stress the ligaments and elicit point tenderness and pain if ligament injuries are present.

Lumbar spine injuries

The lumbar spine, or lower back, is an area that is

subjected to many types of stresses and forces during athletic as well as nonathletic activity. The lower back is very susceptible to injury, and athletes frequently complain of pain in this area. The majority of low back pain in athletes is caused by either acute trauma or chronic stresses.

Occasionally, low back pain is caused by structural defects in the vertebrae or intervertebral discs. All conditions affecting the lumbar spine can be aggravated by various contributing factors, such as inadequate or inappropriate conditioning, inflexibility, congenital anomalies, of poor postural habits.

Each of these factors should be kept in mind when evaluating injuries to the lumbar spine area. The most common athletic injuries to the lower back are contusions, sprains, and strains. Contusions are more common in the paraspinal muscles but may also occur over the subcutaneous spinous processes.

The athlete will often have a history of a direct blow to the lumbar area, with localized tenderness and pain on movement. Sprains and strains are common in the multiplicity of muscles and ligaments in the lower back. Both of these injuries can be caused by the same types of mechanisms and may occur simultaneously.

Violent muscle contractions against resistance, overuse, and overstretching are the most common mechanisms resulting in sprains or strains in the soft tissues along the spine. The complex anatomy of the lower back makes it very difficult to stress and evaluate specific muscles and ligaments.

As a result, it is difficult to differentiate between a spring and strain in this area. Fortunately, it is also usually unnecessary, as both of these injuries are treated symptomatically. Severe injuries to the lumbar spine, such as fractures or dislocations, are extremely rare in athletic activity. Neurologic damage as a result of such an injury is also not as likely as in the cervical spine because the spinal cord ends at about the first lumbar vertebrae and the peripheral nerves in the cauda equina are more mobile and resistant to trauma.

Compression fractures, as previously described in the thoracic spine, can also occur to the bodies of the lumbar vertebrae. However, the most common fractures in the lower back involve the spinous or transverse processes. These can occur as a result of a direct blow or violent muscle contraction. Fractures of this type are at times indistinguishable from severe strains or confusions without radiographs. The most common structural defect of the lumbar spine in athletes is a condition called spondylolysis, which is a defect in the pars interarticularis of the vertebrae.

If this defect is bilateral, it may allow that vertebrae to slip forward on the vertebra or sacrum below, a condition called spondylolisthesis. It may develop in athletes involved in strenuous exercise or competition. Many authorities consider this condition to be a stress fracture and the result of repeated trauma and stress rather than an acute fracture.

It is also believed that spondylolysis and spondylolisthesis can be congenital. The athlete with spondylolisthesis will usually complain of low back pain associated with increased activity. With rest or inactivity the pain diminishes, only to return again once activity is resumed.

In addition to the pain in the lower back, the athlete may complain of pain radiating into the buttocks and upper thighs. The appearance of radiating pain, as well as recurrent episodes of low back pain with activity, should alert the athletic trainer to refer this athlete for further diagnosis and radiographs. Occasionally the pain level remains tolerable and the athlete continues activity without ever knowing about the spondylolisthesis.

Sacrum and Coccyx

The sacral and coccygeal portions of the spine are often referred to as the false, or fixed, vertebrae. Together, the sacrum and coccyx form the terminal portion of the spinal column. In addition, they form the strong wedge shaped posterior portion of the bony pelvis.

Numerous ligaments of the sacrum and coccyx attach to portions of the lumbar vertebrae above and to points on the bony pelvis laterally and below. The sacrum is a large wedge-shaped structure formed by the fusion of five vertebrae . The inner surface of the sacrum is smooth and concave, whereas the outer surface is convex, and rough.

The upper portion articulates with the body of the fifth lumbar vertebra, and the lower portion articulates with the coccyx below. The concave inner surface is grooved by four transverse ridges that show the points of separation between the original bodies of the five sacral vertebrae before fusion.

At each end of the transverse ridges are large openings, which accommodate the sacral nerves and arteries. The prominent sacral promontory is a bony prominence projecting from the anterior border of the base. The coccyx forms the body tip of the spine.

It is generally a single, triangular bone fused from four rudimentary vertebrae. These vertebrae are very small and consist of only the fused body and poorly developed transverse processes. No laminae or spinous processes are present. Occasionally, the first element, or vertebrae, in the coccyx may be separate from the rest.

The upper portion of the coccyx, called the base, articulates with the sacrum. The coccyx diminishes in size until it reaches the tip. Athletic injuries to the coccyx are not common but may occur from a direct blow to the area, such as a kick or a fall to a sitting position. Although these injuries may be painful, they generally are not disabling and require only routine treatment procedures.

Sacroiliac Joints

The sacroiliac joint is formed by the articulation between the sacrum and the iliac portion of the hip bones on each side of the pelvis. It is true synovial joint but movement is limited by the presence of interlocking facets of bone and by extremely strong and dense ligaments.

Any appreciable movement in either or both of the sacroiliac joints would lead to gross instability in the erect posture. In the sitting or standing position, the full weight of the body above the pelvis passes through these joints.

Therefore freedom of motion must be sacrificed for stability. The sacrum hangs from the sacroiliac joints and is kept from being pushed forward into the pelvis by the interlocking facets of bone and by the posterior sacroiliac ligaments, which are the strongest in the body

The dimple on each side immediately above the buttock is a useful external surface landmark that defines the centre of the sacroiliac joint in most young adults. True sacroiliac sprains are extremely rare and almost never occur as a result of athletic activity.

ATHLETIC INJURY ASSESSMENT PROCESS

The potential for spinal injuries resulting in neurologic damage such as permanent paralysis or death is present in most athletic activities, especially contact sports. With any injury involving the spine, it is extremely important for the athletic trainer to recognize the possibilities for neurologic involvement as quickly as possible.

Selection of appropriate assessment procedures, handling manoeuvres, and transportation techniques depends on the possibility of involvement of the spinal cord. Added neurologic damage can occur during improper positioning or movement of an injured athlete. At no time in the assessment of athletic is the principle "do not harm" more important than when evaluating and caring for injuries involving the spine. Athletes suffering an injury to the spine generally present themselves is one of two modes.

The athlete may suffer a traumatic injury and remain lying on the court or field. In these instances the injured athlete should be treated as though he or she has sustained a serious spinal cord injury until proved otherwise. This includes protecting the injured athlete from any unnecessary movement during the assessment process until you can be sure there is no spinal cord involvement. It is more common, however, for the athlete with an injury to the back or neck to be moving about.

Primary Surgery

The primary surgery is of utmost importance when an injured athlete remains down and appears to be unresponsive or unconscious. Maintenance of airway, breathing, and circulation must then by primary considerations. Remember, whenever a neck injury is suspected, movement of the cervical spine must not occur.

If the athlete is unconscious and a neck injury is suspected, the jaw-thrust method of opening the airway is the safest technique to use. If the injured athlete must be moved to perform CPR techniques, it is extremely important that he or she be rolled or moved as a unit to avoid any unnecessary movements of the spine. After assurance that the respiratory and circulatory states of the injured athlete are adequate, proceed to the secondary survey and a more detailed neurologic evaluation.

Secondary Surgery

The evaluation procedures used during the secondary surgery depend on the responsiveness and position of the injured athlete. A quick glance at the overall picture will generally determine the direction in which the athletic trainer will proceed with the secondary surgery. It is important to maintain a high index of suspicion whenever assessing spine injuries, as there may be associated damage to the spinal cord or peripheral nerve roots.

TREATMENT

A spinal cord trauma is a medical emergency requiring immediate treatment to reduce the long-term effects. The time between the injury and treatment is a critical factor affecting the eventual outcome.

Corticosteroids, such as dexamethasone or methylprednisolone, are used to reduce swelling that may damage the spinal cord. If spinal cord compression is caused by a mass (such as a hematoma or bony fragment) that can be removed or brought down before there is total destruction of the nerves of the spine, paralysis may in some cases be reduced or relieved. Ideally, corticosteroids should begin as soon as possible after the injury.

Surgery may be necessary. This may include surgery to remove fluid or tissue that presses on the spinal cord (decompression laminectomy). Surgery may be needed to remove bone fragments, disk fragments, or foreign objects or to stabilize fractured vertebrae (by fusion of the bones or insertion of hardware).

Bedrest may be needed to allow the bones of the spine, which bears most of the weight of the body, to heal.

Anatomic realignment is important. Spinal traction may reduce dislocation and/or may be used to immobilize the spine. The skull may be immobilized with tongs (metal braces placed in the skull and attached to traction weights or to a harness on the body).

Treatment will address muscle spasms, care of the skin, and bowel and bladder dysfunction.

Extensive physical therapy, occupational therapy, and other rehabilitation interventions are often required after the acute injury has healed. Rehabilitation assists the person in coping with disability that results from spinal cord trauma.

Spasticity can be reduced by many oral medications, medications that are injected into the spinal canal, or injections of botulinum toxins into the muscles. It is important to treat pain with analgesics, muscle relaxants, or physical therapy modalities.

Core Stabilization Program

Low back pain will affect 80% of the population. And, although the pain may go away after 4 to 6 weeks, the deep stabilizing muscles of the lower back will remain impaired. Impaired deep stabilizing muscles provide poor segmental stiffness, and this predisposes your back to re-injury and a return of lower back pain.

Using a stabilizer, a biofeedback and gym ball for strengthening the back muscles and to improve the stability of spine. This is a proven effective technique to strengthen deep spinal muscles.

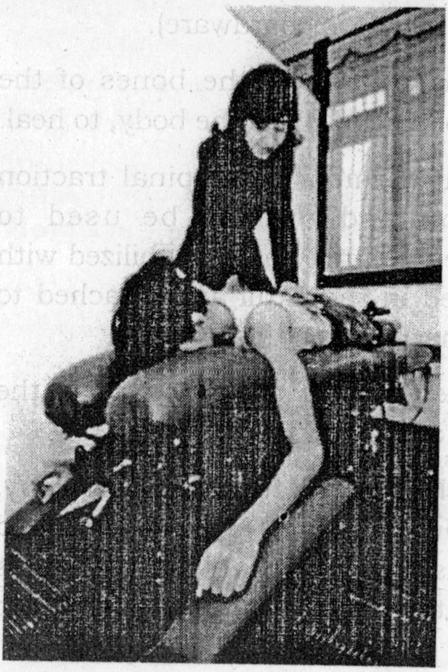

Manual Therapy and Mobilization

Spinal mobilization has a significant role to play in the treatment of neck and back pain particularly where restricted mobility is present. Restoration of spinal mobility, both in physiological movement and in vertebral segmental mobility, often results in a reduction in the patient's pain and spasm.

Spinal Decompression (DTS) Therapy for Neck/Back Pain

This is a specialized treatment targeting disc herniation or prolapsed disc - Utilizing the DTS System (Chattanooga-USA) to create negative intra-discal pressure and relieve the symptoms of back and leg pain or neck and arm pain.

DTS Therapy provides relief of pain from back, sciatica, pinched nerve, neck and degenerated /

herniated disc disease. During this treatment, by cycling through distraction and relaxation phases a spinal disc can be isolated and placed under negative pressure, causing a vacuum effect within it.

Studies verify the significant reduction of intradiscal pressures into the negative range, to approximately - 150 mm/HG, which result in the non-surgical decompression of the disc and nerve root. Conventional traction has never demonstrated a reduction of intradiscal pressure to negative ranges; on the contrary - many traction devices actually increased intradiscal pressure, most likely due to reflex muscle spasm. The Decompression Table is designed to apply distraction tension to the patient's lumbar /cervical spine without eliciting reflex contractions of the paraspinal muscles.

How does it work?

Treatment

DTS Therapy is performed on a specially designed table in either a face up or face down position. You will be comfortably positioned on the table and fitted with a harness attached to the computer controlled traction which is programmed to deliver a gentle stretching force to the spinal vertebra. These scientifically designed DTS pull patterns are designed to facilitate anti-inflammatory effect for healing, Decompressive effect on disc, and Spinal mobilization effect for reducing stiffness. The treatment time is between 15-25minutes.

Vacuum or pumping effect

The gentle stretching and relaxing of the spine causes a pumping action that promotes nutrition intake into the discs, something often lost in damaged and degenerative disc conditions. In healthy discs this occurs naturally with movements and body positions. An injured or degenerated disc gets fewer nutrients and hydration. Stretching the spine in a controlled manner can help re-establish a more normal pumping action to re-supply the disc with nutrients and blood to help the disc heal. This also creates negative pressure in the disc (decompression) that can help the drawing in of a bulge and help take pressure off a "pinched" spinal nerve.

Core muscle strength and conditioning

Most patients feel significant pain reduction in as few as five DTS treatments. That however does not mean the healing process is complete, or that your pain won't return. So when pain is under control we need to focus on rehabilitating the structures supporting the disc in order to fully heal your discs and keep the pain from returning. To improve spine flexibility and increase muscle control is vital for spinal health.

A program of focused rehabilitative exercise, with Stabilizer Pressure Biofeedback may begin during or after your DTS Therapy course of treatment. Through a series of specific slow moving and controlled exercise techniques (often targeting the abdominal muscles); the Biofeedback monitors the correctness and effectiveness of your exercise performance. It provides you with continual visual feedback and ensures you a quality and precise exercise session. Studies show consistent stabilization and endurance exercises control back pain and reduce injury.

Long term pain relief

Regular and consistent home-based exercise is one of the keys to long-term relief. Post treatment you will be taught a home-based exercise program that will help to bring your spine back to full health. This exercise program may include postural advice, Stabilizer/ Exercise ball exercises and resistance training and other "core" exercises.

What other treatment is involved in addition to the Spinal Decompression Therapy?

In addition to the DTS itself treatment may include any of the following therapies as indicated by your condition: - electrical stimulation therapy, ultrasound therapy, ice / heat therapy, laser therapy, spinal mobilization and active rehabilitation exercises.

How often do I take the treatment?

It depends on the complexity and extent of rehabilitation needed .DTS is usually performed 3-5 times a week for 15-20 sessions and your response is continually evaluated. Further treatments may be necessary or a reduced frequency may be recommended at that time.

11

Head Injuries

Head Injury Overview

Head injury is a general term used to describe any trauma to the head, and most specifically to the brain itself.

Skull fracture: A skull fracture is a break in the bone surrounding the brain and other structures within the skull.

Linear skull fracture: A common injury, especially in children. A linear skull fracture is a simple break in the skull that follows a relatively straight line. It can occur after seemingly minor head injuries (falls, blows such as being struck by a rock, stick, or other object; or from motor vehicle accidents). A linear skull fracture is not a serious injury unless there is an additional injury to the brain itself.

Depressed skull fractures: These are common after forceful impact by blunt objects-most commonly, hammers, rocks, or other heavy but fairly small objects. These injuries cause "dents" in the skull bone. If the depth of a depressed fracture is at least equal to the thickness of the surrounding skull bone (about 1/4-1/2 inch), surgery is often required to elevate the bony pieces and to inspect the brain for evidence of injury. Minimally depressed fractures are less than the thickness of the bone. Other fractures are not depressed at all. They usually do not require surgical treatment unless other injuries are noted.

Basilar skull fracture: A fracture of the bones that form the base (floor) of the skull and results from severe blunt head trauma of significant force. A basilar skull fracture commonly connects to the sinus cavities. This connection may allow fluid or air entry into the inside of the skull and may cause infection. Surgery is usually

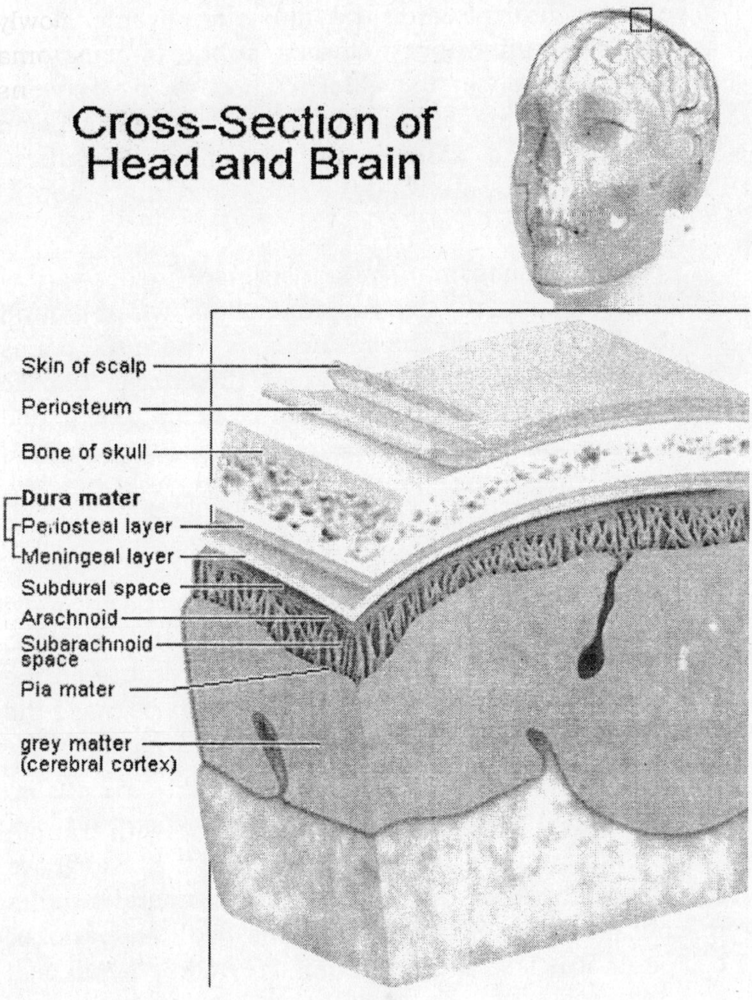

not necessary unless other injuries are also involved.

Intracranial (inside the skull) hemorrhage (bleeding)

Subdural hematoma: Bleeding between the brain tissue and the dura mater (a tough fibrous layer of tissue between the brain and skull) is called a subdural hematoma. The stretching and tearing of "bridging veins" between the brain and dura mater causes this type of bleeding. A subdural hematoma may be acute, developing suddenly after the injury, or chronic, slowly accumulating after injury. Chronic subdural hematoma is more common in the elderly whose bridging veins are often brittle and stretched and can more easily begin to slowly bleed after minor injuries. Subdural hematomas are potentially serious and may require surgery.

Epidural hematoma: The skull is made up of a variety of bones; the dura, the thick membrane that wraps around the brain, attaches at the suture lines where the bones come together. If bleeding occurs in the enclosed space between the dura and the bone, and a hematoma (blood clot) forms, there is nowhere for it to accumulate and pressure within the epidural space can build quickly. The increasing pressure pushes the hematoma against the brain tissue and may cause significant damage.

Tiny epidural hematomas potentially may be observed without surgery, but often surgery is indicated to removed the hematoma and relieve the pressure on the brain. The earlier the operation, the better, because the death rate increases if the patient is in a coma at the time of operation.

An epidural hematoma may often occur with trauma to the temporal bone located on the side of the head above the ear. Aside from the fact that the temporal bone is thinner than the other skull bones (frontal, parietal, occipital), it is also the location of the middle meningeal artery that runs just beneath the bone. Fracture of the temporal bone is associated with tearing of this artery and may lead to an epidural hematoma.

Subarachnoid hemorrhage: Subarachnoid hemorrhage can be caused by trauma and often does not require surgery. Blood accumulates in the space beneath the arachnoid layer that surrounds the brain. While this can irritate the brain and cause symptoms of headache, vomiting, and stiff neck, treatment may be watchful waiting without surgery unless symptoms worsen.

Intraparenchymal hemorrhage/cerebral contusion: These terms describe bleeding into the brain tissue itself. A contusion is like a bruise to the brain tissue and usually requires no special intervention, much like a concussion. Most doctors admit people with cerebral (brain) contusion to the hospital for observation since there may be rare complications such as brain swelling. An intraparenchymal hemorrhage is a pool of blood within the brain tissue. Minor bleeding may stop without any treatment and cause no serious problems. More serious or large bleeds usually require surgery.

Closed head injuries: This broad term describes any injury to the brain or structures within the skull that is not caused by a penetrating injury (such as a gunshot wound or stab wound). They range from very minor to potentially fatal injuries.

HEAD INJURY CAUSES

All types of head injuries can be caused by trauma. In adults in the United States such injuries commonly result from motor vehicle accidents, assaults, and falls. In children falls are the most common cause followed by recreational activities such as biking, skating, or skateboarding. A small but significant number of head injuries in children are from violence and abuse.

Penetrating trauma: Missiles such as bullets or sharp instruments (such as knives, screwdrivers, or ice picks) may penetrate the skull. The result is called a penetrating head injury. Penetrating injuries often require surgery to remove debris from the brain tissue. The initial injury itself may cause immediate death, especially if from a high-energy missile such as a bullet.

Blunt head trauma: These injuries may be from a direct blow (a club or large missile) or from a rapid deceleration force (a fall or striking the windshield in a car accident).

HEAD INJURY SYMPTOMS

Signs and symptoms of head injuries vary with the type and severity of the injury.

Minor blunt head injuries may involve only symptoms of being "dazed" or brief loss of consciousness. They may result in headaches or blurring of vision or nausea and vomiting. There may be longer lasting subtle symptoms including, irritability, difficulty concentrating, insomnia, and difficulty tolerating bright light and loud sounds. These post concussion symptoms may last for a prolonged period of time.

Severe blunt head trauma involves a loss of consciousness lasting from several minutes to many days or longer. Seizures may result. The person may suffer from severe and sometimes permanent neurological deficits or may die. Neurological deficits from head trauma resemble those seen in stroke and include paralysis, seizures, or difficulty with speaking, seeing, hearing, walking, or understanding.

Penetrating trauma may cause immediate, severe symptoms or only minor symptoms despite a potentially life-threatening injury. Death may follow from the initial injury. Any of the signs of serious blunt head trauma may result.

WHEN TO SEEK MEDICAL CARE

Emergency personnel should immediately attend to all potentially serious head injuries.

Call the doctor to ask about any of the following situations. Your doctor will recommend home care, set up an appointment to see you, or direct you to go to a hospital's Emergency Department.

- A person is pushed to the ground or struck a hard object with the head but did not lose consciousness
- Vomiting more than once
- Confusion
- Drowsiness
- Weakness or inability to walk

Severe headache

Go to the Emergency Department by ambulance in the following situations. People with less severe injuries may be taken by car to the Emergency Department.

- Severe head trauma or a fall from more than the height of the person or a hard fall onto a hard surface or object
- Loss of consciousness for more than 1 minute, vomiting more than once, confusion, drowsiness, weakness or inability to walk, or severe headache
- Prevent movement of the neck in severe head injury or if the injured person has any neck pain. If the person needs to vomit, carefully roll them onto their side without

turning the head.

• Should an injured person be allowed to fall asleep? Many people mistakenly believe that it is important to keep a person awake after they have been struck on the head. Children often are more emotionally disturbed than they are physically injured after a minor fall. They will cry and be upset, but as the parent rushes them to the hospital, the child may begin to calm down. They have expended a lot of physical and emotional energy by crying and then will often want to fall asleep.

• You do not need to keep a child or other victim of head injury awake. In many cases it is even helpful to the emergency doctor to be able to awaken a child who is now calm and rested and able to behave normally. This gives the doctor a much better assessment of the severity of the head injury.

• If a person who was initially normal after a head injury cannot be awakened or is extremely difficult to awaken, he or she may have a more serious head injury and should be evaluated by a doctor.

HEAD INJURY TREATMENT

Self-Care at Home

Emergency medical personnel should immediately treat any serious or potentially serious head injury.

Minor head injuries may be cared for at home.

Bleeding under the scalp, but outside the skull, creates "goose eggs" or large bruises at the site of a head injury. They are common and will go away on their own with time. Using ice immediately after the trauma may help decrease their size.

Do not apply ice directly to the skin. Ice should be applied for 20-30 minutes at a time and can be repeated about every 2-4 hours as needed.

Use a light washcloth as a barrier and wrap the ice in it. You can also use a bag of frozen vegetables wrapped in cloth. This conforms nicely to the shape of the head.

Make your own ice pack by adding 1/3 cup of 70% isopropyl alcohol (the green-colored kind is best to help identify it later) to 2/3 cup of water in a zip-lock-style bag (double bag it to prevent leaking). The mixture turns into "slush." Freeze this homemade ice pack for use when needed. Caution: If you have small children in your home, watch them carefully when using the ice pack. Drinking the mixture can be poisonous.

Commercially available ice packs use chemicals to create cold. They are designed to be kept in a first-aid kit and need not be kept frozen. These can be applied directly to the skin, although a barrier can also be used if bleeding is present. They must be disposed of after a single use but can be handy in case of emergencies.

When a minor head injury results from a fall onto carpet or other soft surface and the height of the fall is less than the height of the person who fell and there is no loss of consciousness (in other words, the person was not "knocked out"), a doctor's visit is not usually needed. Apply ice to lessen swelling.

MEDICAL TREATMENT

Treatment varies widely depending on the type and severity of injuries.

- Minor head injuries are often treated at home as long as someone is available to watch the person.

- Bed rest, fluids, and a mild pain reliever, for example, acetaminophen (Tylenol) may be prescribed. Ice may be applied to the scalp for pain relief and to decrease swelling.

• Cuts will be numbed with a medication usually given by injection. They will then be cleansed. The doctor will then look for foreign matter and hidden injuries. The wound usually is closed with skin staples, stitches (sutures), or skin glue. Tetanus immunization will be updated if needed.

• People with serious closed head injuries are almost always admitted to the hospital for observation and repeated studies to assure that the condition does not worsen.

• Occasionally a head injury may cause elevated pressure within the skull. An intracranial pressure (ICP) monitor probe may be surgically inserted into the brain through the skull to measure the pressure. If the pressure rises too high, it may be necessary to do surgery to decompress the brain. Death is possible. Intravenous medications may be used to control intracranial pressure as a temporizing measure until the crisis resolves or surgery is performed.

• Medication to prevent seizures may be given to prevent or treat seizures that occur from the head injury. Seizures after head injury often do not require treatment because they may not reoccur.

• Antibiotics are usually not required in closed head injuries. Some doctors use antibiotics in all cases of basilar skull fracture. Other doctors do not feel this is useful.

• When there is a closed head injury with bleeding inside the skull, the doctor must consider a number of factors to determine the correct treatment. Some of these include the location of the bleeding, severity of the symptoms, the presence of any other injuries, and progression of symptoms. Surgery may be needed. Other options include pressure monitors, medication to prevent seizures, and antibiotics to prevent infection. People with this type of injury may need a breathing tube inserted (intubation) to help prevent further brain injury. Angiography may be performed.

• Penetrating head injuries often require some sort of surgery, usually to remove foreign material or to stop bleeding. Other options include pressure monitors, medication to prevent seizures, and antibiotics to prevent infection. People with this type of injury may need a breathing tube inserted. Angiography may be performed.

NEXT STEPS

Prevention

• Sensible prevention includes wearing helmets when bike riding, inline skating, driving motorcycles, and other similar activities.

• Safety belts, car seats, and airbags when used properly can prevent head injuries in motor vehicle accidents.

• Drinking while driving is one of the most common causes of motor vehicle crashes. Many serious head injuries would be prevented by avoiding this dangerous behavior.

• Fall-proofing includes checking your home for areas where someone may fall: stairs, bathtubs, throw rugs, and furniture.

12

Hip and Pelvic Injuries

Hip pain in the young athlete can be a diagnostic and treatment dilemma for the clinician. In the past decade, progress in imaging and operative techniques have provided tools to better outfit the orthopedist involved in the care of these patients. Hip pain can be intra-articular or extra-articular, and it is important to distinguish between the two. The differential diagnosis for extra-articular hip pain includes apophyseal avulsion fractures, snapping iliotibial band over the greater trochanter, snapping hamstring over the ischial tuberosity, psoas snapping, psoas tendonitis, hip pointer, and even inguinal hernia. Intra-articular pathology includes all intracapsular sources of pain, including femoral neck stress fracture, ligamentum teres pathology, labral tears, chondral injuries, loose bodies, and slipped capital femoral epiphysis. The treating physician should be aware of pediatric conditions such as hip dysplasia and Legg–Calve Perthes disease, which can predispose the patient to hip pain as adolescents. Although many young patients may be treated with nonoperative means for their hip pain, the physician should be aware of new hip arthroscopic techniques that may be appropriate for their patients.

The runner is especially at risk for development of injury to the hip and pelvis secondary to chronic repetitive microtrauma. The key to treatment is establishing complete and accurate diagnosis, and, in particular, identifying the functional biomechanical deficits in the kinetic chain that contribute to this repetitive microtrauma. A long-term successful outcome and prevention of reinjury are more likely if the focus of rehabilitation is on the restoration of the functional kinetic chain, rather than on a specific injured tissue. For example, the typical treatment of "iliotibial band syndrome" is a stretching protocol that frequently is unsuccessful in the long-term improvement of symptoms. A functional biomechanical approach might identify that the injured runner has lack of calcaneal eversion and a structurally rigid supinated foot. These functional biomechanical deficits would lead to inadequate internal rotation of the tibia and femur and result in inhibition or decreased recruitment of the gluteal muscles, in particular the gluteus medius. Restoring pronation throughout the lower extremity would require joint play techniques or functional joint mobilizations for the foot and ankle. In addition, a running shoe with a cushioned heel may be necessary to promote pronation and to attenuate shock. Exercises that integrate foot and hip function, including balance reaches, lunges and step-downs, are prescribed to stimulate the gluteus medius and other gluteals in positions that simulate running. Activities that are done in this manner activate the entire functional kinetic chain of muscles and joints. The nonoperative sports medicine specialist, in particular the physiatrist and physical therapist, are in an excellent position to integrate treatment of the entire functional kinetic chain through a thorough biomechanical evaluation and comprehensive rehabilitation of the injured runner. Additional training in the areas of biomechanical evaluation and functional biomechanical deficits should be sought, because residency and even many fellowship-trained programs often overlook these important areas. Finally, the injured runner is best taken care of in a setting in which different sports medicine specialists are available and work well as a team. No one sports medicine specialist can provide all of the needs to the injured runner.

HIP FRACTURE TREATMENT

Hip fractures are treated in one of two ways: Traction or orthopedic surgery.

Non-operative treatment

If operative treatment is refused or the risks of surgery are considered to be too high the main emphasis of treatment is on pain relief. Skeletal traction may be considered for long term treatment. Aggressive chest physiotherapy is needed to reduce the risk of pneumonia and skilled nursing to try to avoid pressure sores and DVT/pulmonary embolism Most patients will be bedbound for several months.

Operative treatment

Most hip fractures are treated by orthopedic surgery, which involves implanting an orthosis. The surgery is a major stress on the patient, particularly in older people. Pain is significant, forcing the patient to remain immobilized. Since prolonged immobilization can be more of a health risk than the surgery itself, post-op patients are encouraged to become mobile as soon as possible, often with the assistance of physical therapy (physiotherapy).

Surgery for fractured neck of femur

Fracture treated with cannulated screwsFor low-grade fractures (Garden types 1 and 2), standard treatment is fixation of the fracture in situ with screws or a sliding screw/plate device. This treatment can also be offered for displaced fractures after the fracture has been reduced.

In elderly patients with displaced fractures many surgeons prefer to undertake a Hemiarthroplasty, replacing the broken part of the bone with a metal implant. The advantage is that the patient can mobilize without having to wait for healing.

Surgery for intertrochanteric fracture

Fracture supported by dynamic hip screwAn intertrochanteric fracture, below the neck of the femur, has a good chance of healing. Treatment involves stabilizing the fracture with a lag screw and plate device to hold the two fragments in position. A large screw is inserted into the femoral head, crossing through the fracture; the plate runs down the shaft of the femur, with smaller screws securing it in place.

The fracture typically takes 3–6 months to heal. As it is only common in elderly, removal of the dynamic hip screw is usually not recommended to avoid unnecessary risk of second operation and the increased risk of re-fracture after implant removal. The most common cause for hip fractures in the elderly is osteoporosis; if this is the case, treatment of the osteoporosis can well reduce the risk of further fracture. Only young patients tend to consider having it removed; the implant may function as a stress riser, increasing the risk of a break if another accident occurs.

Prognosis post operation

Among those affected over the age of 65, 40% are transferred directly to long-term care facilities, long-term rehabilition facilities, or nursing homes; most of those affected require some sort of living assistance from family or home-care providers. 50% permanently require walkers, canes, or some other such device for mobility;

all require some sort of mobility assistance throughout the healing process.

Among those affected over the age of 50, approximately 25% die within the next year due to complications such as blood clots (deep venous thrombosis, pulmonary embolism), infections, and pneumonia.[citation needed]

Patients with hip fractures are at high risk for future fractures including hip, wrist, shoulder, and spine. After treatment of the acute fracture, the risk of future fractures should be addressed. Currently, only 1 in 4 patients after a hip fracture receives treatment and work up for osteoporosis the underlying cause of most of the fractures. Current treatment standards include the starting of a bisphosphonate to prevent future fracture risk by up to 50%.

Complications

Complications of the injury

Nonunion, failure of the fracture to heal, is common (20%) in fractures of the neck of the femur, but much more rare with other types of hip fracture. The rate of nonunion is increased if the fracture is not treated surgically to immobilize the bone fragments.

Malunion, healing of the fracture in a distorted position, is very common. The thigh muscles tend to pull on the bone fragments, causing them to overlap and reunite incorrectly. Shortening, varus deformity, valgus deformity, and rotational malunion all occur often because the fracture may be unstable and collapse before it heals. This may not be as much of a concern in patients with limited independence and mobility.

Avascular necrosis of the femoral head occurs frequently (20%) in fractures of the neck of femur, because the blood supply is interrupted. It is rare after intertrochanteric fractures.

Hip fractures rarely results in neurological or vascular injury.

Surgical complications

Deep or superficial wound infection has an approximate incidence of 2%. It is a serious problem as superficial infection may lead to deep infection. This may cause infection of the healing bone and contamination of the implants. It is difficult to eliminate infection in the presence of metal foreign bodies such as implants. Bacteria inside the implants are inaccessible to the body's defence system and to antibiotics. The management is to attempt to suppress the infection with drainage and antibiotics until the bone is healed. Then the implant should be removed, following which the infection may clear up.

Implant failure may occur; the metal screws and plate can break, back out, or cut out superiorly and enter the joint. This occurs either through inaccurate implant placement or if the fixation does not hold in weak and brittle bone. In the event of failure, the surgery may be redone, or changed to a total hip replacement.

Mal-positioning: The fracture can be fixed and subsequently heal in an incorrect position; especially rotation. This may not be a severe problem or may require subsequent osteotomy surgery for correction.

General medical complications

Many of patients are unwell before breaking a hip; it is not uncommon for the break to have been caused by a fall due to some illness, especially in the elderly. Nevertheless, the stress of the injury, and a likely surgery, does increase the risk of medical illness including heart attack, stroke, and chest infection.

Blood clots may result. Deep venous thrombosis (DVT) is when the blood in the leg veins clots and causes pain and swelling. This is very common after hip fracture as the circulation is stagnant and the blood is hypercoagulable as a response to injury. DVT can occur without causing symptoms. A pulmonary embolism (PE) occurs when clotted blood from a DVT comes loose from the leg veins and passes up to the lungs. Circulation to parts of the lungs are cut off which can be very dangerous. Fatal PE may have an incidence of 2% after hip fracture and may contribute to illness and mortality in other cases.

Mental confusion is extremely common following a hip fracture. It usually clears completely, but the disorienting experience of pain, immobility, loss of independence, moving to a strange place, surgery, and drugs combine to cause or accentuate dementia.

Urinary tract infection (UTI) can occur. Patients are immobilized and in bed for many days; they are frequently catheterised, commonly causing infection.

Prolonged immobilization and difficulty moving make it hard to avoid pressure sores on the sacrum and heels of patients with hip fractures. Whenever possible, early mobilization is advocated; otherwise, alternating pressure mattresses should be used.

HAMSTRING INJURY

A Hamstring injury is common in sports. Hamstring injuries are sometimes known as a 'pulled Hamstring'. The term 'pulled muscle' comes from the description of how the injury takes place. Usually the Hamstring muscle is forcibly stretched beyond its limits and the muscle tissue becomes torn. A tear in the Hamstring muscle is referred to as a Hamstring strain and depending on its severity it is classified as a first, second or third degree strain.

Early Hamstring injury treatment consists of the RICE protocol - rest, ice and compression and elevation (never apply ice directly to the skin). Depending upon the severity of the injury, the leg must be rested from sporting activity for between several weeks and several months.

A Hamstring injury is common in sports. Hamstring injuries are sometimes known as a 'pulled Hamstring'. The term 'pulled muscle' comes from the description of how the injury takes place. Usually, the Hamstring muscle is forcibly stretched beyond its limits and the muscle tissue becomes torn. A tear in the Hamstring muscle is referred to as a Hamstring strain by medical professionals and depending on its severity it is classified as a first, second or third degree strain:

1. a first degree strain is damage to a few muscle fibres,

2. a second degree strain is damage to a more extensive number of muscle fibres,

3. a third degree strain is a complete rupture of the muscle itself.

Common Hamstring Injury Signs & Symptoms:

1. A sudden sharp pain in the Hamstring.

2. Pain when stretching the Hamstring.

3. Hamstring pain during a resisted muscle contraction.

What you can do

1. Consult a sports injury expert

2. Apply ice packs to relieve pain

3. Apply compression bandage to control bleeding & swelling

4. Use resistance bands for muscle strengthening

exercises

5. Wear Compression Shorts or thigh support for reassurance during rehabilitation and retain muscle warmth for injury prevention

6. Warm up before sporting activities

7. Cool down following sporting activities

8. Stretch regularly to maintain muscle length

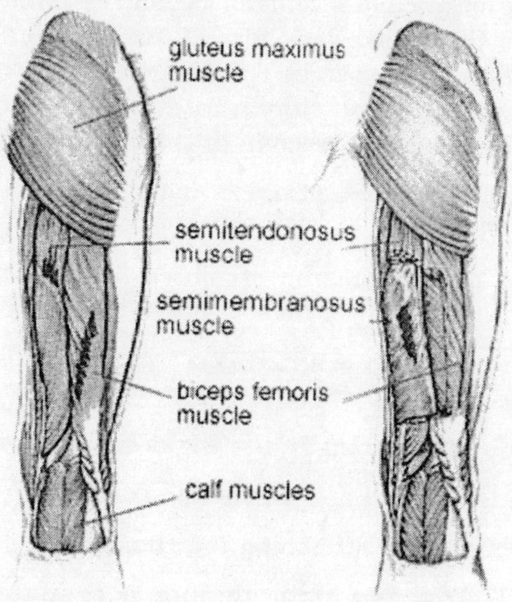

9. Replenish carbohydrates during sporting activity with energy bars & gels

HAMSTRING INJURY SIGNS & SYMPTOMS

With a grade one Hamstring strain the signs may not be present until after the activi+y is over. There may be a sensation of Hamstring cramp or Hamstring tightness and a slight feeling of pain when the muscles are stretched or contracted.

With a grade two Hamstring strain there is immediate pain which is more severe than the pain of a grade one injury. It is confirmed by pain on stretch and contraction of the muscle. A grade two Hamstring strain is usually sore to touch.

A grade three Hamstring strain is a very serious injury. There is an immediate burning or stabbing pain and the athlete is unable to walk without pain. The muscle is completely torn and there may be a large lump of muscle tissue above a depression where the tear is. After a few days with grade two and three injuries a large bruise will appear below the injury site caused by the bleeding within the tissues.

HAMSTRING INJURY TREATMENT

What you can do

1. Consult a sports injury expert

2. Apply ice packs to relieve pain

3. Apply compression bandage to control bleeding & swelling

4. Use resistance bands for muscle strengthening exercises

5. Wear Compression Shorts or Thigh Support for reassurance during rehabilitation

The immediate treatment of a Hamstring muscle injury consists of the RICE protocol - rest, ice, compression and elevation (never apply ice directly to the skin). This is aimed at reducing the bleeding and damage within the Hamstring muscle tissue. Resting may be the common sense approach, but it is one that is often ignored by competitive athletes. This is unwise, since it does not take much to turn a grade one Hamstring strain into a grade two, or a grade two

Hamstring strain into a grade three. As a general rule, grade one Hamstring strains should be rested from sporting activity for about 3 weeks and grade two injuries for about 4 to 6 weeks. In the case of a complete rupture, the Hamstring muscle will have to be repaired surgically and the rehabilitation afterwards will take about 3 months.

Regardless of the severity of the Hamstring injury the treatment in the first few days is the same. The Hamstring should be rested in an elevated position with an Ice Pack applied for twenty minutes every two hours, if practical (never apply ice directly to the skin). A Compression Bandage should be applied to limit bleeding and swelling in the tissues. After the early stages have been spent resting, more active rehabilitation can be started.

Gentle resistance exercises and stretching are important as they help to align the scar tissue that forms during the healing process. By aligning the scar tissue along the normal lines of stress the tensile strength of the Hamstring is enhanced.

At first gentle resistance is provided by a therapist, but as the muscle gets stronger then Resistance Bands can provide more of a challenge. The sets and repetitions are gradually increased and eventually Core Strengthening can be started.

Core Strength and Core Stability exercises can improve muscle function across the trunk and pelvis and this can reduce the risk of Hamstring injury. Core strength exercises on a mat using a Swiss Ball and resistance bands are ideal. Once Core Strength and Hamstring strength are improved, then a return to functional activity is possible. With a grade one Hamstring strain gentle jogging can be initiated between seven and nine days after injury and straight line sprinting is usually started after 3 weeks. Many people find that Warm Pants (Compression Shorts) or a Thigh Support provide reassurance during this active rehabilitation.

Guide to Core Strengthening

Hamstring Injury Prevention

What you can do

1. Warm up before sporting activities
2. Cool down following sporting activities
3. Stretch regularly to maintain muscle length
4. Replenish carbohydrates during sporting activity with energy bars & gels
5. Wear Compression Shorts or Thigh Support to retain muscle warmth

The following measures may have the effect of reducing the risk of sustaining a Hamstring muscle strain:

Warm up prior to matches and training is thought to decrease muscle stretch injuries because the muscle is more extensible when the tissue temperature has been increased by one or two degrees. A good warm up should last at least 20 minutes - starting gently and finishing at full pace activity. Practising sport specific activities helps tune coordination and prepare mentally for competition. Warm Pants (Compression Shorts) or a Thigh Support can be helpful for retaining muscle tissue temperature, ensuring that the tissue remains extensible even in colder weather.

Professional Warm Up Guide

Recovery after training sessions and matches can be enhanced by performing a cool down. This is thought to help muscles get rid of waste products. This is also the ideal time to do stretching exercises.

Professional Cool Down Guide

Maintaining good muscle strength and flexibility may help prevent muscle strains. Muscle strength allows a player to carry out match activities in a controlled manner and decreases the uncoordinated movements which can lead to injury. Tight muscles are associated with strains. Stretching sessions using a Gym Mat can be helpful to maintain muscle length and prevent injury.

Guide to Stretching Exercises

Diet can have an affect on muscle injuries. If a player's diet is high in carbohydrate in the 48 hours before a match there will be a adequate supply of the energy that is necessary for muscle contractions. However, if the muscles become short of fuel, fatigue can set in during training or matches. This fatigue can predispose a player to injury. Carbohydrate can be replenished during training and matches by taking Energy Bars and Gels.

HIP LABRUM TEAR INJURY

Hip pain may be due to a tear of the Acetabular Labrum. The Acetabular Labrum is a fibrocartilage ring, located in the socket (Acetabulum) of the hip joint. The Hip Labrum helps to increase the stability of the hip joint, acting as a 'spacer' and shock absorber during weight bearing. The Acetabular Labrum can become torn if there is a twisting movement while the hip joint is bearing weight, and this hip injury may occur during sports such as soccer and rugby.

The onset of hip pain is usually immediate. As with all hip joint problems, the pain may be diffuse and difficult to pinpoint. If the front of the hip joint is affected there may be a pinching sensation when the person flexes the hip by bringing the knee up to the chest. The pain may be reproduced in sport during activities that require weight bearing and twisting.

Treatment usually involves hip arthroscopy that can be performed on an outpatient basis. Although a general anaesthetic is used, a stay in hospital is not usually necessary. Following a short period on crutches, the patient follows a program of exercises under the supervision of a Chartered Physiotherapist. A return to sports is usually possible between two and three months after the operation.

Common Hip Labrum Tear signs & symptoms:

1. A history of twisting on the hip.
2. Diffuse hip pain.
3. Hip joint 'catching' on specific movements.

What you can do

1. Consult a sports injury expert
2. Use a buoyancy belt for mobilisation exercises in a swimming pool
3. Use resistance bands for muscle strengthening exercises
4. Wear Compression Shorts for reassurance following surgery

HIP ARTHRITIS (OSTEOARTHRITIS)

Hip Arthritis (Osteoarthritis) is a common cause of hip pain and hip stiffness that usually manifests itself in middle age. Hip arthritis is characterised by progressive hip joint degeneration that may be due to hip overuse or secondary to a hip injury such as a Labrum tear.

Damage to the hip joint surfaces can be as a result of sporting trauma, but is more commonly due to repetitive stresses over a long period of time. This is usually associated with habitual overuse of a joint for occupational or sporting purposes. In most individuals, the signs and symptoms do not appear until middle age, but the disease process starts much earlier and the arthritis process can be accelerated following trauma to the hip joint.

Hip pain is the most universal symptom of hip arthritis. This hip pain can be felt around the groin, but may also radiate down the thigh or up to the back. As the arthritis worsens and muscle wasting occurs there is often a pronounced limp. Eventually hip replacement surgery may be required where there is severe hip pain, although hip exercises and physical therapy rehabilitation are very helpful.

Common Hip Arthritis signs & symptoms:

1. History of previous hip injury or hip surgery.
2. Hip pain related to overdoing activities.
3. Hip stiffness, particularly in cold weather.

What you can do

1. Consult a sports injury expert
2. Wear Compression Shorts for therapeutic warmth
3. Use a buoyancy belt for mobilisation exercises in a swimming pool
4. Use resistance bands for Gluteal muscle strengthening exercises
5. Use Shock Absorbing Insoles to reduce stress on the hip
6. Apply ice packs to relieve pain
7. Use anti-inflammatory gel to relieve pain

13

Hand, Wrist and Finger Injuries

At one time or another, everyone has had a minor injury to a finger, hand, or wrist that caused pain or swelling. Most of the time our body movements do not cause problems, but it's not surprising that symptoms develop from everyday wear and tear, overuse, or an injury.

Finger, hand, or wrist injuries most commonly occur during:

- Sports or recreational activities.
- Work-related tasks.
- Work or projects around the home, especially if using machinery such as lawn mowers, snow blowers, or hand tools.
- Accidental falls.
- Fistfights.

The risk of finger, hand, or wrist injury is higher in contact sports, such as wrestling, football, or soccer, and in high-speed sports, such as biking, in-line skating, skiing, snowboarding, and skateboarding. Sports that require weight-bearing on the hands and arms, such as gymnastics, can increase the risk for injury. Sports that use hand equipment such as ski poles, hockey or lacrosse sticks, or racquets also increase the risk of injury.

In children, most finger, hand, or wrist injuries occur during sports or play or from accidental falls. Any injury occurring at the end of a long bone near a joint may injure the growth plate (physis) and needs to be evaluated.

Older adults are at higher risk for injuries and fractures, because they lose muscle mass and bone strength (osteopenia) as they age. They also have more problems with vision and balance, which increases their risk of accidental injury.

Most minor injuries will heal on their own, and home treatment is usually all that is needed to relieve symptoms and promote healing.

SUDDEN (ACUTE) INJURY

An acute injury may occur from a direct blow, a penetrating injury, or a fall, or from twisting, jerking, jamming, or bending a limb abnormally. Pain may be sudden and severe. Bruising and swelling may develop soon after the injury. Acute injuries include:

- **Bruises.** After a wrist or hand injury, bruising may extend to the fingers from the effects of gravity. See a picture of a bruise (contusion).
- **Injuries to ligaments.** See a picture of a torn thumb ligament as in skier's thumb.
- Injuries to tendons, such as mallet finger.
- Injuries to joints (sprains).
- Pulled muscles (strains).
- Broken bones (fractures), such as a wrist fracture.
- Dislocations.
- Crushing injury, which can lead to compartment syndrome.

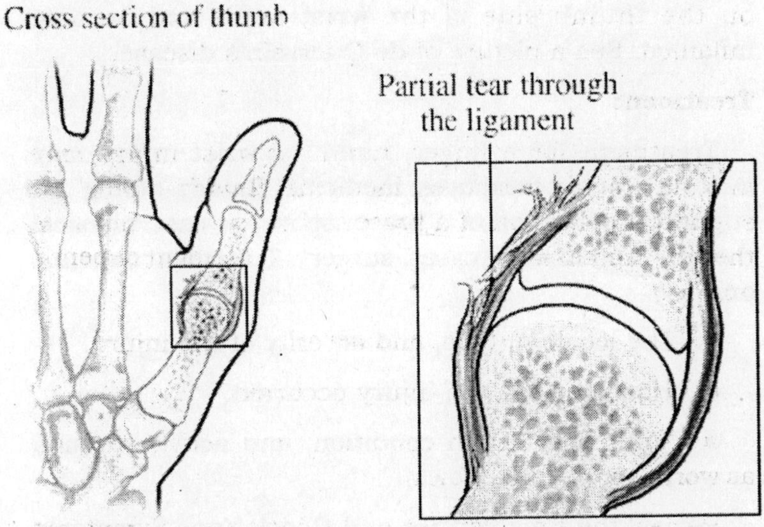

OVERUSE INJURIES

Overuse injuries occur when too much stress is placed on a joint or other tissue, often by "overdoing" an activity or repeating the same activity. Overuse injuries include the following:

- **Carpal tunnel syndrome** is caused by pressure on a nerve (median nerve) in the wrist. The symptoms include tingling, numbness, weakness, or pain of the fingers and hand. See a picture of carpal tunnel syndrome.

- **Tendon pain** is actually a symptom of tendinosis, a series of very small tears (microtears) in the tissue in or around the tendon. In addition to pain and tenderness, common symptoms of tendon injury include decreased strength and movement in the affected area.

- **De Quervain's disease** can occur in the hand and wrist when tendons and the tendon covering (sheath) on the thumb side of the wrist swell and become inflamed. See a picture of de Quervain's disease.

Treatment

Treatment for a finger, hand, or wrist injury may include first aid measures; medicine; "buddy-taping" for support; application of a brace, splint, or cast; physical therapy; and in some cases, surgery. Treatment depends on:

- The location, type, and severity of the injury.
- How long ago the injury occurred.
- Your age, health condition, and activities (such as work, sports, or hobbies).

Review the Emergencies and Check Your Symptoms sections to determine if and when you need to see a doctor.

Emergencies

Do you have any of the following symptoms that require emergency treatment? Call 911 or other emergency services immediately.

- Signs of shock occur:
- In children.
- In adults and older children.
- Severe bleeding does not slow during the first 15 minutes of steady, direct pressure.
- Any part of your hand is partially or completely amputated. Begin first aid measures.
- Pieces of bone are visible in a wound, or a bone is sticking through the skin. Note: Do not try to push the bone back into the skin. Cover the area with a clean bandage.

- Injection of a substance under high pressure into the hand, such as paint from a high-pressure paint sprayer or a nail from a powered nail gun

- Severe pain with pale, white, blue, or cold fingers or hand

Check Your Symptoms

If you answer yes to any of the following questions, click on the "Yes" in front of the question for information about how soon to see a health professional.

Review health risks that may increase the seriousness of your symptoms.

If you have any of the following symptoms, evaluate those symptoms first.

- **Bleeding:** Go to the topic Cuts or Scrapes.

- Puncture wound or injection of a foreign body under high pressure: Go to the topic Puncture Wounds.

- A finger, hand, or wrist problem not related to an injury: Go to the topic Finger, Hand, and Wrist Problems, Noninjury.

- Injury from cold exposure: Go to the topic Cold Temperature Exposure.

- A burn to a finger, hand, or wrist: Go to the topic Burns.

- A bite to a finger, hand, or wrist: Go to the topic Animal and Human Bites.

- A fingernail problem or blood under a nail: Go to the topic Nail Problems and Injuries.

HOME TREATMENT

First aid for a suspected broken bone

- If a bone is sticking out of the skin, do not try to

push it back into the skin. Cover the area with a clean bandage.

- **Control bleeding.**

- Remove all bracelets or rings. It may be difficult to remove the jewelry once swelling occurs, which in turn can cause other serious problems, such as nerve compression or restricted blood flow. See a picture of removing a ring that is stuck.

- Free a trapped finger or hand from an object, such as a pipe, toy, or jar.

- Splint the injured area without trying to straighten the injured limb. Loosen the wrap around the splint if signs develop that indicate the wrap is too tight, such as numbness, tingling, increased pain, swelling, or cool skin below the wrap. A problem called compartment syndrome can develop.

- Home treatment for a sore or sprained finger

- Use rest, ice, compression, and elevation (RICE) for pain and swelling.

- If you do not have diabetes or peripheral arterial disease, your sore or sprained finger can be " buddy-taped" to your uninjured finger next to it. Protect the skin by putting some soft padding, such as felt or foam, between your fingers before you tape them together. Your injured finger may need to be buddy-taped for 2 to 4 weeks to heal. If your injured finger hurts more after you have buddy taped it, remove the tape and use the Check Your Symptoms section to check your symptoms again. Caution: Never splint a finger in a completely straight position, such as on a Popsicle stick. For proper healing, the finger should be slightly bent and in a relaxed position.

- Stop, change, or take a break from activities that

cause your symptoms.

- Home treatment for a minor hand or wrist injury

- Home treatment may help relieve pain, swelling, and stiffness.

- Remove all rings, bracelets, or any other jewelry that goes around a finger or wrist. It will be more difficult to remove the jewelry later if swelling increases.

- Use rest, ice, compression, and elevation (RICE) for pain and swelling.

- Do not use your injured hand or wrist for the first 24 hours after an injury, if possible. An elastic bandage can help decrease swelling. The wrap will also remind you to rest the injured hand or wrist. A wrist splint can help support an injured wrist. Talk to your doctor if you think you need to use a splint or bandage for more than 48 to 72 hours.

- Gently massage or rub the area to relieve pain and encourage blood flow. Do not massage the injured area if it causes pain.

- For the first 48 hours after an injury, avoid things that might increase swelling, such as hot showers, hot tubs, hot packs, or alcoholic beverages.

- After 48 to 72 hours, if swelling is gone, apply heat and begin gentle exercise with the aid of moist heat to help restore and maintain flexibility. Some experts recommend alternating between heat and cold treatments.

- Treat blisters.

Safety tips

- Be sure to follow these safety tips when you use a nonprescription medicine:

- Carefully read and follow all directions on the medicine bottle and box.
- Do not take more than the recommended dose.
- Do not take a medicine if you have had an allergic reaction to it in the past.
- If you have been told to avoid a medicine, call your doctor before you take it.
- If you are or could be pregnant, do not take any medicine other than acetaminophen unless your doctor has told you to.
- Do not give aspirin to anyone younger than age 20 unless your doctor tells you to.
- Symptoms to Watch For During Home Treatment
- Use the Check Your Symptoms section to evaluate your symptoms if any of the following occur during home treatment.
- Pain or swelling develops.
- Signs of infection develop.
- Numbness; tingling; or cool, pale skin develops.
- Symptoms do not improve with home treatment.
- Symptoms become more severe or frequent.

Prevention

The following tips may prevent finger, hand, and wrist injuries.

- Do exercises that strengthen your hand and arm muscles.
- Stop, change, or take a break from activities that cause your symptoms.
- Reduce the speed and force of repetitive

movements in activities such as hammering, typing, knitting, quilting, sweeping, raking, playing racquet sports, or rowing.

- Change positions when holding objects, such as a book or playing cards, for any length of time.
- Use your whole hand to grasp an object. Gripping with only your thumb and index finger can stress your wrist.
- Consider wearing gloves that support the wrist and have vibration-absorbing padding when working with tools that vibrate.
- Use safety measures, such as gloves, and follow instructions for the proper use of hand and power tools.
- Use caution when using knives in preparing food or craft activities. Supervise a child using knives or sharp scissors in craft activities.
- Wear protective gear, such as wrist guards, in sports activities.
- Review your work posture and body mechanics.
- Organize your work so that you can change your position occasionally while maintaining a comfortable posture.
- Position your work so you do not have to turn excessively to either side.
- Keep your shoulders relaxed when your arms are hanging by your sides.
- When using a keyboard, keep your forearms parallel to the floor or slightly lowered and keep your fingers lower than your wrists. Allow your arms and hands to move freely. Take frequent breaks to stretch your fingers, hands, wrist, shoulders, and neck. If you

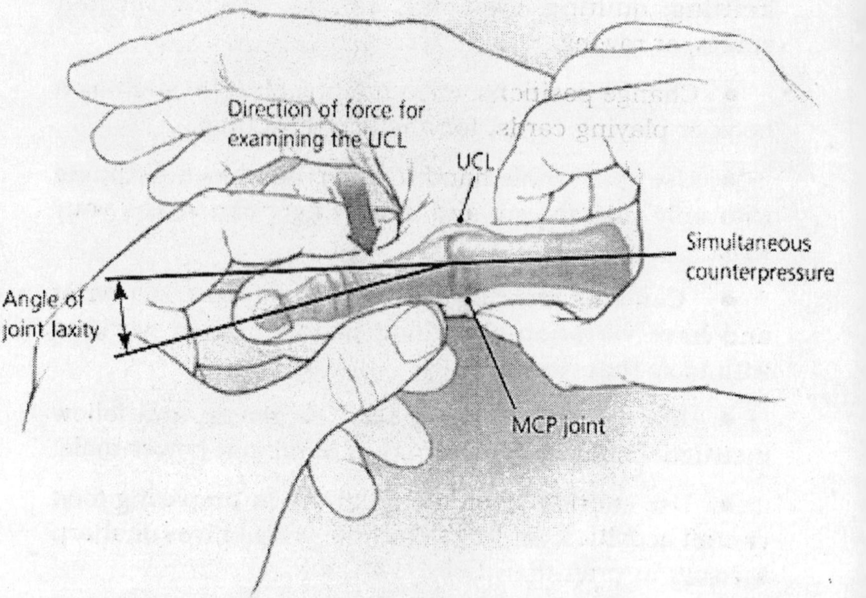

use a wrist pad during breaks from typing, it's best to rest your palm or the heel of your hand on the support, rather than your wrist.

Reduce Falls

- Take steps to prevent falls and injuries in adults, such as removing any obstacles from your walking path.
- Take steps to prevent falls and injuries in babies and toddlers, such as not leaving your baby unattended in any infant seat or "sitting" toy.

General Prevention Tips

- Wear your seat belt in a motor vehicle.
- Don't carry objects that are too heavy.

- Use a step stool. Do not stand on chairs or other unsteady objects.

- Wear protective gear during sports or recreational activities, such as roller-skating or soccer. Supportive splints, such as wrist guards, may reduce your risk for injury.

- Warm up well and stretch before any activity. Stretch after exercise to keep hot muscles from shortening and cramping.

- Use the correct techniques (movements) or positions during activities so that you do not strain your muscles.

- Avoid overusing your hand and wrist doing repeated movements that can injure your bursa or tendon. In daily routines or hobbies, examine activities in which you make repeated arm movements.

- Consider taking lessons to learn the proper techniques for sports. Have a trainer or person who is familiar with sports equipment check your equipment to see if it is well-suited for your level of ability, body size, and body strength.

- If you feel that certain activities at your workplace are causing pain or soreness from overuse, talk to your human resources department for information on alternative ways of doing your job or to discuss equipment modifications or other job assignments.

Keep Your Bones Strong

- Eat a nutritious diet with enough calcium and vitamin D, which helps your body absorb calcium. Calcium is found in dairy products, such as milk, cheese, and yogurt; dark green, leafy vegetables, such as broccoli; and other foods.

- Exercise and stay active. It is best to do weight-bearing exercise (walking, jogging, stair climbing, dancing, or lifting weights) for 45 to 60 minutes at least 4 days a week. Weight-bearing exercises stimulate new bone growth by working the muscles and bones against gravity. Exercises that are not weight-bearing, such as swimming, are good for your general health but do not stimulate new bone growth. Talk to your doctor about an exercise program that is right for you. Begin slowly, especially if you have been inactive. For more information, see the topic Fitness.

- Don't drink more than 2 alcoholic drinks a day if you are a man, or 1 alcoholic drink a day if you are a woman. People who drink more than this may be at higher risk for weakening bones (osteoporosis). Alcohol use also increases your risk of falling and breaking a bone.

- Do not smoke or use other tobacco products. Smoking puts you at a much higher risk of developing osteoporosis. It also interferes with blood supply and healing. For more information, see the topic Quitting Tobacco Use.

Jammed Finger

A jammed finger is a frustrating sports injury. It can happen in just about any sport, and while seemingly simple, can really put a damper on your ability to play. Learn more about finger sprains, how they happen, and what to do about them below.

What is a Jammed Finger?

A jammed finger, in medical terms, is a sprain of the joint capsule of the inter-phalangeal joints. What? In English? It is injury to the knuckles.

A joint sprain involves injury to ligaments or the joint capsule. Every joint in the body is comprised of both ligaments and joint capsule in order to connect the bones together. The fingers, although often overlooked, are no different. Just like other joints, the capsule and ligaments can be damaged if subjected to significant force...which leads us to how a jammed finger happens...

Jamming Your Finger

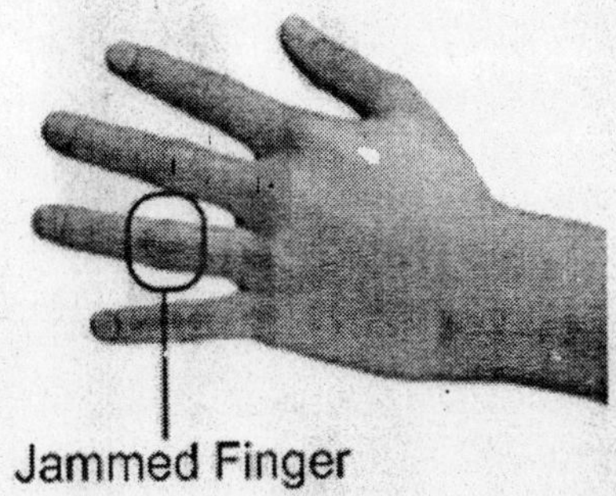

It has probably happended to you before. You were reaching out to catch the basketball, and it moved funny, or you weren't quite ready, and it caught you right on the end of your finger. It hurts like crazy, and kinda stuns you for a minute. That is how you jam your finger.

The force that hits the end of the finger is translated through the bones into the joint. Often, the ends of the phalanges (finger bones) are bruised at the knuckle, and this is what causes the swelling, as well as damage to the capsule.

There are other ways to suffer a finger sprain. You can get it bent the wrong way, or too far another way. You can get it stepped on, smashed between two helmets, hit with a baseball, or any other numerous ways that produce enough force to cause injury. Fingers are in the middle of most sports, and they tend to get hurt.

Symptoms of a Jammed Finger

Pain, swelling, loss of motion, and loss of strength are all very common symptoms of a jammed finger. Swelling within the joint is very obvious, and you can usually tell very easily when you have suffered a finger sprain.

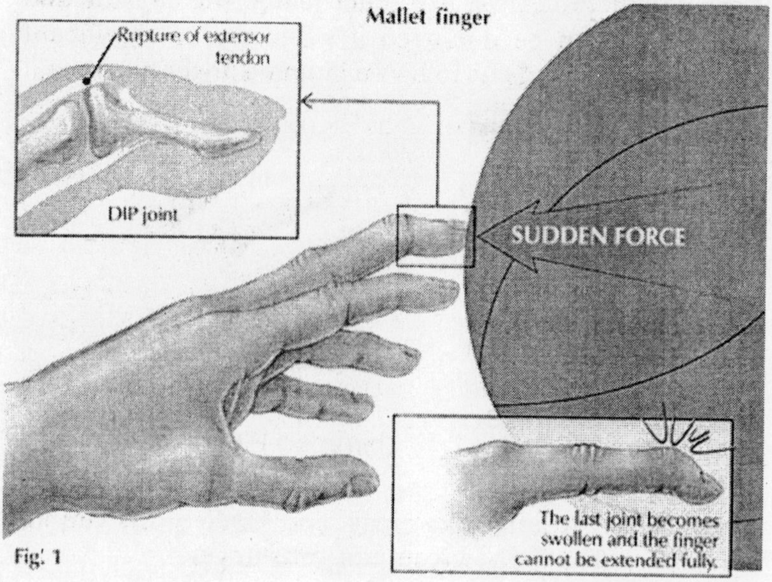

Fig. 1

One knuckle will swell up, and it will look noticibly bigger than the others. Unfortunately, this swelling often lasts for weeks if not months. Sometimes it never completely goes away.

Pain and motion usually come back fairly quickly, depending on how severe the sprain is.

Treating a Jammed Finger

Treating pain and swelling are the first steps of treating a jammed finger. As soon after injury as you can, use the R.I.C.E. Principles to help reduce your pain and discomfort. Depending on how much pain, swelling, and loss of motion you have, you may need to see your physician.

This is especially true if you took a pretty hard hit to the finger, or if it was bent backwards violently. You may have suffered a finger fracture and not just a sprain. It is sometimes hard to differentiate between the two, so an

X-ray may be a good idea to be safe.

Once a fracture is ruled out, you can begin working on improving your range of motion and strength. Use ice and rest for a few days, and then begin trying to bend and straighten the finger. Do this gently, only pushing into mild discomfort. Gradually, your motion will return, as swelling goes down.

Some finger sprains may need to be splinted. If you have significant swelling and pain, see your physician, and they will direct you with treatment.

Summary

Jammed fingers are very common in sports, and they are ofen overlooked as insignificant. This is sometimes true, but a little rest and ice can go a long way to reduce the time it takes to heal, and to get things back to normal.

Don't assume that you just sprained your finger. If you have lots of swelling and pain, see your physician for an X-ray. Fingers, although overlooked, are extremely important to your sports participation, and in the rest of life. Do yourself a favor and take care of them.

14

Stress Fractures

A stress fracture is one type of incomplete fracture in bones. It is caused by "unusual or repeated stress". This is in contrast to other types of fractures, which are usually characterized by a solitary, severe impact.

It could be described as a very small sliver or crack in the bone; this is why it is sometimes dubbed "hairline fracture". It typically occurs in weight-bearing bones,

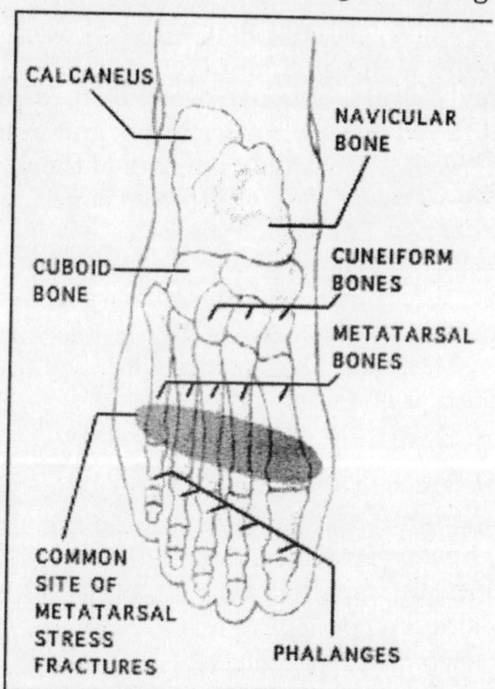

such as the tibia (bone of the lower leg) and metatarsals (bones of the foot).

It is a common sports injury, and most cases are associated with athletics.

Presentation

Stress fractures usually have only a few symptoms. A stress fracture could present as a generalized area of pain and tenderness associated with weight bearing. Usually when running, a stress fracture in the leg or foot will cause severe pain at the beginning of the run, moderate pain in the middle of the run, and severe pain at the end and after the run.

Diagnosis

As with most conditions, a stress fracture is best diagnosed after interview and examination by a physician. Investigations are not necessary to diagnose a stress fracture.

X-rays usually do not show any evidence of stress fractures, so a CT scan, MRI, or 3-phase bone scan may be more effective in unclear cases.

Treatment

If a stress fracture occurs in a weight-bearing bone, healing will be delayed or prevented by continuing to put weight on that limb.

Rest is the only option for complete healing of a stress fracture. The amount of recovery time varies greatly depending upon the location, severity, and the strength of the body's healing response. Complete rest and a cast or walking boot are usually used for a period of four to eight weeks, although periods of rest of twelve to sixteen weeks is not uncommon for more severe stress fractures. After this period a very gradual resuming of activities may be resumed, as long as the activity does not cause pain. While the bone may feel healed and not hurt during daily activity, the process of bone remodeling may take place for many months after the injury feels healed, and incidences of re-fracturing the bone is still at significant risk. Activities such as running or sport that place additional stress on the bone should only gradually be resumed. One general rule is to not increase the volume of training by more than 10 percent from one week to the next.

Rehabilitation usually includes muscle strength training to help dissipate the forces transmitted to the bones.

Bracing or casting the limb with a hard plastic boot or air cast may also prove beneficial by taking some stress off the stress fracture. An air cast has pre-inflated cells that put light pressure on the bone, which promotes healing by increasing blood flow to the area. This also reduces pain because of the pressure applied to the bone. If the stress fracture of the leg or foot is severe enough, crutches can help by removing stress from the bone.

With severe stress fractures, surgery may be needed for proper healing. The procedure may involve pinning the fracture site, and rehabilitation can take up to a half year.

Causes

Bones are constantly attempting to remodel and repair themselves, especially during a sport where extraordinary stress is applied to the bone. Over time, if enough stress is placed on the bone that it exhausts the capacity of the bone to remodel, a weakened site—a stress fracture—on the bone may appear. The fracture does not appear suddenly. It occurs from repeated traumas, none of which is sufficient to cause a sudden break, but which, when added together, overwhelm the osteoblasts that remodel the bone.

Stress fractures commonly occur in sedentary people who suddenly undertake a burst of exercise (whose bones are not used to the task). They may also occur in Olympic-class athletes who do extraordinary quantities of high-impact exercise, in professional and amateur distance runners who run high weekly mileage, or in soldiers who march long distances.

Muscle fatigue can also play a role in the occurrence of stress fractures. Consider a human runner. With each stride, large forces are exerted at various places in the legs. Each shock — a rapid acceleration and energy transfer — must be absorbed. Both muscles and bones serve as shock absorbers. However, the muscles, usually those in the lower leg, become fatigued after running a long distance and lose their ability to absorb shock. As the bones now experience larger stresses, this increases the risk of fracture.

Previous stress fractures have been identified as a risk factor.

Frequency

Dr Johnathan C Reeser states that, in the US, the annual incidence of stress fractures ranges from 5% to 30%, depending on the sport and other risk factors. Stress fractures occur less frequently in those of black African descent than in Caucasians, due to a generally higher BMD (bone mineral density) in the former. Women and highly active individuals are also at a higher risk. The incidence probably also increases with age due to age-related reductions in BMD. But children may also be at risk because their bones have yet to reach full density and strength. The female athlete triad also can put women at risk, as disordered eating and osteoporosis can cause the bones to be severely weakened.

Prevention

One method of avoiding stress fractures is to add more stress to the bones. Though this may seem counter-intuitive (because stress fractures are caused by too much stress on the bone), moderate stress applied to the bone in a controlled manner can strengthen the bone and make it less susceptible to a stress fracture. An easy way to do this is to follow the runner's rule of increasing distance by no more than 10 percent per week. This allows the bones to adapt to the added stress so they are able to withstand greater stress in the future.

Strengthening exercises also help build muscle strength in the legs. Strengthening these muscles will prevent them from becoming fatigued quickly, allowing them to absorb the strain of running for longer periods of time. Key muscles that need strengthening with lower leg stress fractures are the calves and the shin muscles. Runners often suffer from overuse injuries or repetitive stress injuries. These include stress fractures, stress reactions, tendinitis, meniscal tears, ITB Friction syndrome, and exacerbation of pre-existing arthritis. Stress fractures, if not diagnosed and treated, can develop into complete fractures.

Depending on a variety of factors (including weight, running surface and shoe durability), runners should replace their shoes every 300-700 miles to allow adequate mid-sole cushioning. A change in running surfaces can also help prevent stress fractures. However, it is also argued that cushioning in shoes actually causes more stress by reducing the body's natural shock-absorbing action, increasing the frequency of running injuries.

During exercise that applies more stress to the bones,

it may help to increase calcium and vitamin D intake, depending on the individual. Also, it is important to monitor diet, because nutrition plays a vital role in bone development. Some individuals are at risk of osteoporosis, and depending on the country in which medical care is being supplied, there may be an osteoporosis screening program available.

WHAT IS A STRESS FRACTURE?

A stress fracture is a common overuse injury most often seen in athletes. Usually, a fracture, or broken bone, is caused by an acute event, such as a car crash or a fall. When this is the case, the bone experiences a very high force that causes the stress fracture.

A stress fracture occurs when the forces are much lower, but happen repetitively for a long period of time; these injuries are also known as "fatigue fractures." Stress fractures are commonly seen in athletes who run and jump on hard surfaces, such as distance runners, basketball players, and ballet dancers.

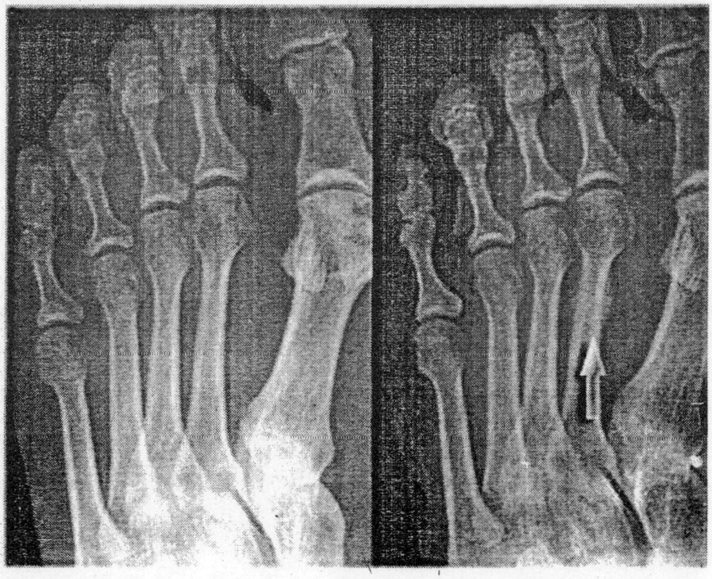

A stress fracture can occur in any bone, but is commonly seen in the foot and shin bones. They rarely occur in the upper extremity because the weight of your body is not supported by your arms as it is in your legs.

How is a stress fracture diagnosed?

Physical examination and history are important in diagnosing stress fractures. Because these overuse injuries have a typical course and common physical findings, the history and examination can be critical in the diagnostic evaluation. X-Rays usually do not show a stress fracture, but they may show evidence of bone attempting to heal around the stress fracture. Further studies, including an MRI or bone scan may be necessary if the diagnosis is unclear or if the problem does not resolve with treatment.

Bone is constantly undergoing changes to adapt to its environment. When astronauts go into space, they are known to develop a thinning of the bone similar to osteoporosis. The reason is that their skeleton is not under the constant demands of gravity, and the bone adapts to that environment. Stress fractures are usually seen in athletes who increase their level of activity over a short period of time. The increased demand placed on the bone causes the bone to remodel and become stronger in the areas of higher stress. However, if the response of the bone cannot maintain the pace of the repetitive demands, a stress fracture may result.

Another factor that can contribute to the development of a stress fracture are dietary abnormalities and menstrual irregularities. Because both factors contribute to bone health, any problems with diet (e.g. poor nutrition, anorexia, bulimia) or menstruation (amenorrhea) may place an individual at higher risk for these injuries. This is one reason that adolescent female athletes are at particularly high risk for development of a stress fracture.

What is the treatment for a stress fracture?

The best treatment is almost always resting the injured leg. If there is no evidence that the stress fracture may displace, then avoiding the overuse activity may be sufficient treatment. However, if there is a concern of displacement of the stress fracture, then weight-bearing should be avoided (i.e. use crutches), and a cast may be placed. One rule of thumb (but not an absolute rule) is: if there is pain, don't do it. This means if jogging causes pain where you have a stress fracture, don't jog. If walking causes pain in that location, use crutches.

Other general stress fracture treatment principles include:

1. Ice the injured area
2. Wear proper equipment, specifically footwear
3. Increase activities gradually
4. If pain develops and persists, seek medical advice

SUMMARY

Each day, the body makes new bone to replace the bone that is broken down by the stress of everyday living. Usually, this process is balanced, with the body replacing the equal amount of bone lost. However, this balance may become upset. The body, due to several factors, may not produce sufficient bone. As a result, micro cracks, called stress fractures, can occur in the bone.

Factors that my affect the building process are too little sleep, a diet with inadequate calcium, a rapid increase in activity. Sometimes stress fractures may result from minor trauma, like accidentally kicking one leg when running.

How Will I Know If I Have A Stress Fracture?

Stress fractures produce pain in a limited area directly over the point of the bone where the fracture has occurred. The pain is made worse by activity and is improved with rest.

On physical examination, there is pain when pressure is applied to the injured area. Hopping or jumping on a leg with a stress fracture will cause increased pain. Frequently, but not always, there is swelling around the injured area.

X-rays are not usually helpful in diagnosing an early stress fracture because the bones will look normal and the micro cracks are not visible. After several weeks of rest to allow the bone to repair itself, a healing reaction callus can be seen on an X-ray.

The diagnosis of an early stress fracture can usually be confirmed by a bone scan. In this procedure, a substance normally used by the bone for repair is injected into the patient's bloodstream. After 2 or 3 hours, the patient is placed under a scanner to detect the amount of substance distributed throughout the bones. All of the bones will absorb some of the substance, but if a bone is repairing a stress fracture, it will absorb more of it at the fracture site, and will appear darker than the other bones. An MRI may also be used to confirm the diagnosis.

Stress fractures are among the more common injuries that occur usually in sporsperson especially in athletes. They are a source of disability, but that disability is usually brief. With early diagnosis, treatment usually becomes simple and the period of disability is lessened. Thus, it is important that those people caring for runners be aware of the typical history, physical findings, and any laboratory tests that help to make the diagnosis of a stress fracture. The magnitude of the problem is considerable, because it has been estimated that between 4.7% and 15.6% of all injuries to runner are stress fractures. The first medical description of what we now call stress fractures was reported in 1855 and concerned military recruits. During the next 110 years, many reports in the literature described "march" or "fatigue" fractures in military rectuits. Only with the increased awareness of fitness and particularly with the running of fitness and particularly with the running boom, beginning in the 1960s, did these same types of fractures in runners begin to be recognized. At that point, the term stress fracture came into general use. A simple definition of a stress fracture is any bone fracture that does not occur as a result of a single traumatic episode sufficient to cause fracture of the involved bone.

Stress fractures may occur when abnormal stress is applied to normal bone or when normal stress is applied to weekend bone. In either instance, this could result in what we clinically identify as a stress fracture, which fits into the category of the overuse injuries that are so commonly encountered in many athletes but particularly in runners. Stress fractures occur in all sports that require repetitive running and jumping but are far more common in long-distance runners than in any other athletes. A distinct difference is observed in the bony sites where stress fractures occur in military recruits versus the sites in which they occur in runners. A question thus arises about the cause of stress fracture in the two groups or at least about the various factors affecting the production of the fractures. Military recruits are frequently people in relatively poor physical condition who, when they start training, are rapidly made to undertake significant physical fitness activities including running and marching. Both the skeletal and muscular systems are rapidly loaded under the military training system.

Giladi and colleagues reported that changing the military footwear and the training surfaces and using ortotic devices dramatically decrease the incidence of stress fractures in military population. The calcaneus and the metatarsals are the most common sites of stress fractures in military personnel. Metatarsal stress fractures are also noted in runners but far less commonly than those in the tibia, whereas calcaneal stress fractures are uncommon in runners. Runners have the highest incidence of stress fractures for all athletes—more than in all other sports combined—as sown by one large series. Of the 320 stress fractures reported by Matheson and associates, 221 were due to running and the other 90 were due to various other sports, most of which entailed running. In that particular series, the tibia was the most commonly affected bone, being involved 49% of the time, and the weekly running mileage of the afflicted patients ranged from 25 to 44 miles per week.

Causes of Stress Fractures

It is interesting that despite all of the clinical material about stress fractures that has bee voluminous reports in the literature, we do not know the precise cause of stress fractures. A great deal of information shows that frequent running causes an overload to the bony skeleton that in some way subverts the usual dynamic reparative process that we associate with normal bone repair. The amount of running and the time in which this stress is delivered seem to be important. In Sullivan and colleagues' 1983 study of stress fractures in 51 runners, only 5 would have been classified as joggers.

Personal experience and reading the literature

indicate that 20 miles per week is a reasonable cutoff, in the sense that the vast majority of stress fractures occur in people who are running more than 20 miles per week. It appears that the inability of bone to withstand certain stresses is dose related. Under the usual circumstance, normal bone reacts to both direct and muscular stress by an adaptation response called Wolff's law. We know that bone can respond by remodeling, and either too much or too little stress can cause changes in the normal biologic response of bone., The early literature refers only to the direct effect of weight-bearing stress on the bones as being a primary cause of stress fractures. Later reports refer to the effect of muscle forces acting on the bone, particularly in certain areas. In either case, the forces exceed the stress-bearing capacity of the affected bone. Guoping and Cowokers and Johnson have investigated the histology of stress fractures, and their findings have been well summarized by McBryde.

Continued repetitive stress on the bone leads to a normal remodeling response that is gradually overcome, and trabecularmicro fractures occur. Osteoclastic resorption results from accelerated cortical bone remodeling, which should lead to increased periosteal new bone formation and reinforcement. At this point, if the newly formed bone is not strong enough to accept the stress being exerted, the osteoclastic activity continues. At some point, the structural integrity is broached and a stress fracture occurs. Marymont and colleagues, McBryde, and others believe that certain other conditions occurring in runners such as the ubiquitous shin splints, medial tibial stress syndrome, and tibial periostitis are preroentgenographic stress fractures. They believe that these clinical syndromes represent a continuum that, if runners continue to run, would eventuate in the production of a clinical and roentgenographic stress fracture.

How Is A Stress Fracture Treated?

A cast is usually not required for a stress fracture. Unlike a fracture caused by a blow to the body which injures the skin, muscle, and bone, a stress fracture involves only the bone.

If pain occurs while walking, crutches or a cane should be used to keep weight off the injured extremity. Returning to activity will be a gradual process. Swimming or biking, both non-weightbearing activities can be done to maintain cardiovascular and muscle conditioning in the early period after the stress fracture.

Gradually, impact activities like walking can be added. When the patient can walk rapidly without pain, running can be started. Jumping should only be done when running does not cause any pain. A gradual increase of stress to the bone is the key. Each increase in activity should be done slowly and for short amounts of time. After a while, the activities can be done at a higher intensity and a longer duration. Eventually the level of activity can be increase (see charts 1 and 2).

If, when advancing to the next level of intensity, pain occurs, the patient should return to the lower level for several days before trying again. The physician will guide the patient through these steps and can monitor the degree of fracture healing with X-rays.

It should be noted that while the normal amount of calcium required for bone repair is 1500 milligrams in postmenopausal women and 1000 milligrams for all other adults, increasing calcium intake above this level will not help the stress fracture heal more rapidly.

15

Female Athlete Injuries

There has been a marked increase in female athletes since the passage of Title IX in 1972...over a 10 fold increase in just the number of girls participating in high school sports...at all age levels and at all competitive levels. Associated with this increase is a rising number of injuries reported in gymnastics, cheerleading, running, basketball and soccer. Interestingly, the injury rates in high school basketball and soccer are essentially the same in boys and girls...but the injuries are different. Cheerleading has been reported to be "the leading cause of direct fatal and nonfatal injuries among high school and college women.

A report on gymnastic injuries in children was published this week in Pediatrics. Between 1990 and 2005, "an estimated 425,900 children 6 through 17 years of age were treated in US hospital emergency departments for gymnastic - related injuries...averaged 26,600 annually". The highest rates occurred in children 12 to 17 years of age (17.4/1000)...82% were in girls. "Upper extremity fractures/dislocations were most common for children 6 to 11 years of age (50%). Lower extremity sprains/strains were most common for children 12 to 17 years of age (52%)". The majority of children were able to be treated in the emergency department and sent home (97%).

Some other common sports played by girls/women are running, soccer and basketball. They have specific and, in some cases, an even higher rate of injuries including...anterior cruciate ligament (ACL) tears (basketball and soccer), knee cap pain, shin splints and compartment syndrome of the lower leg (runners) as well as plantar fasciitis and the iliotibial band syndrome. A great deal of attention has been paid to ACL injuries by orthopaedic surgeons because the injury is a serious one, surgery is usually required and prevention is ideal. Many reasons have been speculated on why girls/ women are at higher risk than men for ACL tears. Hormonal changes have been largely discounted, but several characteristis are emerging as important risk factors: the wider angle between the hips and knees, "women apparently cut or suddenly change direction differently than men...women change direction on just 1 foot...while men often use 2 feet" according to a sports expert; and when women jump they tend to land with their knees fully extended (straight) while men land with their knees flexed (bent).

These careful observations by sports experts have led to better training techniques and coaching. Female athletes are being coached to learn how "to run, jump, land and twist safely". New training techniques have apparently reduced the number of ACL injuries in female athletes. In addition, strength training is important as are proper sports gear, orthotics, splints, taping and other techniques used by trainers/coaches that help the athlete prevent injury.

It is intended to be a resource for physicians caring for active and athletic women, focuses on the specific problems encountered by women in sports. In giving health care to active women the physician needs to be empathetic, to demonstrate respect for the patient's athleticism, and to be willing to research or refer problems that may be special to the athletic woman. The last thing a woman who participates in sports and athletic activities wants to be told is to curtail her active lifestyle. The patient will rarely do so; instead, the doctor will lose the patient, and the patient will lose the opportunity to receive the information and medical care she needs.

Now-a-days women are taking part in all types of games and competitions and their number is on the rise. The statistics of women taking part in inter-collegiate, national and international competitions presents an encouraging picture.

Women take to sports as do men for improving physical fitness and recreation. This is all the more important for them as they can bear healthy children. Further, women are very conscious of their form and beauty and fat reduction. Their participation in sports meets this requirement.

Notwithstanding all this, due to their constitution, they are discouraged or prohibited from taking up constant sports because they are likely to be easily injured by impact. Women are said to have weak stamina and heart. They are, therefore, not allowed to take up endurance sports. Further, in other sports too some relaxation is made.

The constitution and physiology of women is different from men in certain respects and this poses some problems. In this comes breast, menstruation and pregnancy.

To evaluate the myth that women are weak and unathletic the Armed forces conducted two major studies. The investigators concluded that the gross differences between men and women are primarily the results of traditional sex bias, which, rather than actual physiologic differences, has resulted in women rarely exercising to their potential fitness levels. Furthermore, they noted that the present national fitness standards for women are far below women's true physiological potential.

GYNAECOLOGIC CONCERNS

Menstrual function is not completely understood. It is an orchestration of hormones in the hypothalamus, pituitary, ovaries, thyroid, and adrenal glands. Physical stress, emotional stress, weight loss, change in body fat, exercise, and dietary changes can affect the hormones produced by these glands and thereby alter menstrual function.

The pubertal awakening of gonadotropic hormones is thought to be central in origin, genetically controlled and linked to attainment of critical body weight. In the normal cycle, the hypothalamus synthesizes and releases gonadotropin-releasing hormone. This hormone stimulates the production of two pituitary hormones, follicle-stimulating hormone and luteinizing hormone. In the preovulatory phase, FSH stimulates the graafian follicle to grow. The graafian follicle secretes estrogen, which stimulates the growth of the endometrium. The rising estrogen level stimulates the hypothalamic release of more GnRH, which triggers the surge of FSH and LH, which causes the release of the ovum from the graafian follicle. In the postovulatory phase the graafian follicle, without the ovum, undergoes transformation into the corpus luterum. The corpus luterum secretes large amounts of estrogen and progesterone. The estrogen continues to stimulate the endometrium to grow, and progesterone converts an estrogen-stimulated endometrium into a stable structure necessary for the fertilized ovum to implant.

If a fertilized ovum does not implant, the corpus luteum has a life span of approximately 12 days. It then degenerates and stops producing estrogen and progesterone, and shedding of the endometrial lining begins. A normal menstrual cycle is measured from the first day of menstrual flow in one cycle up to, but not including, the onset of menstrual flow of the following cycle. The normal range is generally considered to be 21 to 36 days. The preovulatory phase begins with the first day of menstrual flow and ends the day before ovulation. The postovulatory phase begins at ovulation and ends before the onset of the next menstrual flow.

Menarche

Some women who begin exercising before puberty have delayed onset of menses. Management of delayed menarche depends on age. If a girl is 14 years old and has not started menstruating but is developing breast, auxiliary and public hair, the treatment is reassurance and follow-up. If at age 14 the girl is not developing secondary sexual characteristics, or at age 16, whether she has secondary sexual characteristics or not, a workup for primary amenorrhea should be initiated. Recent studies suggest there should be concern about an increased incidence of scoliosis and decreased bone mass in young women with delayed puberty.

Definitions. The literature on menstrual cycle abnormalities is often contradictory and contusing. Although the causes of menstrual cycle abnormalities are not always evident, if is important to be aware of the medical consequences.

1. Menstruation is the cyclic, physiologic discharge through the vagina of blood and mucosal tissue from the nonpregnant uterus.

2. A shortened luteal phase—less than 8 days may be due to an inadequate corpus luteum. This may be a reason for infertility.

3. Anovulation is the absence of egg release. The woman may have cyclic or irregular menstrual periods. It is a hormonal state of unopposed estrogen.

4. Oligomenorrhea is a condition in which menstrual cycles occur at intervals longer than 36 days. It may be caused by anovulation.

5. Amenorrhea is the absence of a menstrual cycle. Primary amenorrhea is the failure of menstruation to occur at puberty. Secondary amenorrhea means cessation of menstruation after it has once been established at puberty. There are many accepted definitions of how many cycles must be missed to constitute secondary amenorrhea. In this text it is defined as no menstrual cycle in a consecutive 6-month period.

Significance of Menstrual Irregularities

In an anovulatory cycle the hormonal environment of unopposed estrogen has been associated with endometrial hyperplasia and the risk of cancer of the endometrium and breast. In amenorrhea estrogen is low and progesterone is absent. If amenorrhea is long-standing, the woman is at risk for decreased bone density, atrophic vaginitis, and urethritis.

Prevalence. Reported prevalences of secondary amenorrhea range from 3.4 to 43%, depending on the investigator's definition of amenorrhea and the selection of subjects. The prevalence of exercise-related menstrual changes depends on age, previous menstrual cycles, and the exercise status of the women.

Any woman who is concerned about her menstrual cycle should be evaluated, but the extent of the evaluation will depend on the content of the patient's history. The two most common causes of amenorrhea are pregnancy and situational tress. Prolactin-secreting tumours are not uncommon, especially in women with galactorrhea. Hirsutism may suggest hyperandrogenism. Premature ovarian failure is also part of the differential diagnosis. The pathogenesis of exercise-related oligo/amenorrhea correlates with exercise intensity, exercise duration and type, weight loss and thinness, body composition, age, previous menstrual irregularity, physical stress, emotional stress, and dietary factors.

Contraception

It is amazing how little high school and college students know about contraception and reproduction. Contraception for the active woman is generally the same as that for other women. Ideal methods of birth control do not exist. Current methods include barriers, the diaphragm and spermicidal jelly, condoms, oral contraceptives, tubal ligation, and vasectomy of male partners. Women who are taking the newer low-dose oral contraceptives often ask how they can control when they have their menstrual periods. One can recommend a switch to 1/25's; using one of these formulations, they may add a few pills from another cycle to delay menses.

Infertility

With an athletic couple having difficulty

conceiving, the first recommendations to the woman include decreasing mileage/training and increasing body fat, if the woman is thin. High-intensity long-distance male runners may have lower sperm counts, and therefore the same recommendations apply to them. It should also be recommended that the woman start recording basal body temperature to help evaluate ovulation. Her partner should have a sperm count. It is estimated that 40% of infertility problems can be attributed to a decrease or absence of spermatogenesis. If this program is not successful after 6 months, the usual in fertility workup should be initiated.

Heavy Bleeding

The normal menstrual flow is approximately 40 ml/cycle. One "full tampon or pad" has approximately 3.5 ml of blood. Therefore, if the flow uses more than 8-10 full pads, the individual is at risk for iron-deficiency anaemia. Menorrhagia in endurance athletes is usually due to an anovulatory cycle. Treatment is progesterone withdrawal on days 16-25. If this is not successful, endometrial curettage is warranted. Metrorrhagia warrants endometrial sampling before initiating progestational therapy to rule out hyperplasia or adenocarcinoma of the endometrium.

Breast Examination

Athletic women should be encouraged to perform breast examinations monthly just after the menstrual period. A good support bra should generally be recommended. If painful breasts are a problem, a reduction or avoidance of caffeine and salt should be suggested. Vitamin B_6 and body fat reduction are also helpful. Bromocriptine for fibrocystic breast disease is indicated if symptoms are severe.

PREGNANCY AND WOMEN ATHLETES

Exercise and Pregnancy

Women who exercise and are athletes often come to their family physicians with questions about exercise and pregnancy. Their most pressing concern is usually how exercise will affect the fetus. It is very important to take a careful exercise history. Is the woman just starting an exercise program? Is she a recreational or a high-performance athlete? What are her concerns and desires?

Major areas of concern of the exercising pregnant woman include:

- What is the effect of elevated body temperature on the fetus?
- Will exercise shunt blood from the uterus to the exercising muscle?
- Will the athletic mother's potentially lower body weight and smaller weight gain compromise the fetus?

Lotgering et al., in an exhaustive review of maternal and fetal responses to exercise during pregnancy, conclude that "although the increased demands of pregnancy might compete with those of exercise, under most circumstances the maternal organism can meet the combined demands of gestation and exercise through a remarkable reserve of physiological adjustments. The effects of exercise on pregnancy that must be addressed in counselling the pregnant woman include heat stress, uterine oxygen consumption, and infant size.

Heat Stress and The Fetus

Some studies show that "fetal temperature lags

behind the rapidly changing maternal temperature at the onset and cessation of exercise. Although heat stress has been reported to cause fetal growth retardation, intrauterine death, and central nervous system defects in several species, the effect of heat stress during exercise has not been systematically investigated on a large scale in humans. Jones et al., studied four aerobically conditioned women to characterize the changes in maternal body temperature and het storage as these women continued to exercise with advancing pregnancy. It was found that maternal core temperature and heat storage did not exceed physiologic limits during exercise. Conditioned maternal thermoregulatory mechanisms appear capable of dissipating the heat production by both the metabolically active fetus and the mother during moderate aerobic exercise. The increased maternal plasma volume during pregnancy helps maintain optimal fetomaternal heat transfer and dissipation. It is important to realize that any large-scale study would be difficult, but more research is necessary before this question can be fully answered.

Unterine Oxygen Consumption

Several human and ovine studies have shown that blood is shunted from the uterus to the exercising muscle. Therefore, another major concern is that the fetus may be compromised. Further studies show that because of increased haemoglobin concentration during pregnancy, and thus increased blood oxygen-carrying capacity, and a flow redistribution within the uterus favouring fetal blood flow at the expense of myometrial flow, the fetus is not compromised. Again, more studies need to be done.

Issue of Smaller Babies

In a controlled study, Clapp demonstrated that "women who continued endurance exercise at or above a minimum conditioning level throughout the first, second, and well into the third trimester gained less weight, delivered earlier, and their infants had a consistent reduction in birth weight for gestational age without increased immediate morbidity. The consistent reduction in birth weight was approximately 500 grams. The question is, does being smaller mean being unhealthy? In the past, one criterion used to judge whether a condition had an adverse effect on a pregnancy was to compare the birthweight of the newborn with controls of similar socioeconomic levels. Some authors have used this argument to suggest that exercise is detrimental. Clapp also noticed that the birth weights of infants born to women who exercised intensively only until the 28th week of pregnancy were not reduced compared with those of infants of nonexercising controls.

The Melpomene study of pregnancy and running provides data based on a questionnaire completed by 1995 women. They concluded that only a few health-care providers view running as a positive aspect of a healthy pregnancy, that participants gradually reduce mileage and speed as the pregnancy progresses, and that the average birthweight is 7 ib, 6 oz.

Another indicator or fetal well-being is the non-stress test. In a small study the non stress test was conducted before and after a 1.5-mile jog in the third trimester of pregnancy. All tests were reactive, with no difference in the mean time to obtain a reactive test before exercise compared with after exercise. Exercise did produce a fetal tachycardia of 155-204 bpm compared with baseline heart rates of 140-155, and a mean of 22 minutes was required for the fetal heart rate to return to the pre-jogging baseline. The authors concluded that moderate exercise in pregnancy does not result in acute fetal distress, but they allowed for the possibility that the fetal tachycardia may be compensatory.

The comments and studies quoted in this section are in reference to healthy pregnancies. Any history of heart disease, diabetes, hypertension, a previous miscarriage, incompetent cervix, anaemia, kidney problems, or vaginal bleeding must be evaluated and treated difference. In cardiac patients, especially those with mitral or aortic valve disease, cardiac output decreases during pregnancy, making exercise dangerous.

Benefits of exercise in pregnancy include weight control, improved muscle tone, maintenance of self-esteem, decreased varicose veins, decreased backache, better sleep, and a sense of control when so many physiologic changes are occurring that are not under one's control. Possibly, but not yet prone, exercise may result in easier pregnancy, labour and delivery.

EATING DISORDERS AND WOMEN ATHLETES

Anorexia Nervosa

Physicians treating female athletes should be able to recognize patients with eating disorders. The prevalence of anorexia nervosa, a syndrome of self-imposed starvation and distorted body image, has increased over the past 15 years from 0.1% to nearly 1% of the general American population. In certain athletic activities, such as ballet, gymnastics, and running, the prevalence of eating disorders is much greater.

In appearance some anorexic women are indistinguishable from high-performance athletes. It is essential to make the diagnosis because anorexia nervosa is often fatal.

Anorexia appears to be the product of a complex interaction of biologic, psychologic and socio-cultural factors. The diagnostic criteria for anorexia nervosa are evolving, with the most common thread being a distorted body image. Differentiating athletic anorexic patients from athletes who are striving for low body-fat levels to enhance performance is difficult and often tentative. Twenty-four per cent of anorexic women are intensely athletic. Obtaining a history of disturbed body image, marked feelings of inadequacy, and depression may take time and repeated visits in order to develop a trusting relationship. History should also be obtained from family members.

Treatment must be multifaceted, including medical, behavioural and family therapy, as well as personal psychotherapy—with the immediate concern being return of the patients' nutritional status to normal and the long-term goal, the resolution of the behavioural and pschodynamic processes.

Bulimia

Bulimia is a syndrome of secretive binge-eating episodes followed by self-induced vomiting, fasting, tand purging with laxatives and/or diuretics. The patients are aware that the eating pattern is abnormal and generally maintain weight with frequent fluctuations.

The prevalence among college students has been reported to be as high as 10%. Medical complications in bulimics include extreme amounts of weight reduction and losses of dangerous quantities of fluids and electrolytes. They may also develop dental cries due to erosion of enamel and gums, esophageal tears secondary to vomiting, and acute gastric dilatation.

Weight Loss in Athletes

Excessive weight loss and food aversion in athletes appears to be different from that seen in anorexics and bulimics. In athletes it may be situationally related to athletic performance and/or "making weight." Males and females appear to be at equal risk, affected athletes are recognized relatively early, and the stresses are usually not deep-seated chronic problems but an accumulation of immediate short-term concerns. Frequent counselling visits as well as instructing the athlete to spend mealtimaes in the company of team-mates or friends may be helpful. The prognosis is significantly better than that for anorexia nervisa. Male Analog. A group of compulsive male distance runners was compared to anorectics with the suggestion that they shared basic personality characteristics. The implication was that this form of exercise addiction is a male analog of anorexia nervosa. This view is not universally shared.

MUSCULOSKELETAL PROBLEMS

Are there specific musculoskeletal problems in women and women athletes? Early studies of injuries in women athletes showed a higher incidence of injuries sustained as compared with men, but these studies also reflected the lack of adequate conditioning in women rather than a true physiological weakness and predisposition to injury. Injuries were more sports-specific than gender-specific; that is, injury types and rates were similar for men and women in the same sport but different for women participating in different sports.

Patellofemoral Pain

Female athletes commonly experience retropatellar knee pain. Symptoms include crepitus, aching, pain going up and down stairs, stiffness after sitting for long periods, and sometimes a subjective feeling of instability. In the recent literature this is referred to as patellofemoral stress syndrome rather than chondromalacia patella, which is an actual pathologic softening and fraying of the retropatellar surface.

In the past, this problem was considered to be a female affliction caused by the influence of the broader gynecoid pelvis on the mechanics of the knee. Several recent studies indicate that it is also common among male athletes.

Ligamentous Laxity

The issue of increased ligamentous laxity has been raised as a reason women are more predisposed to ligamentous injuries, but this may have been due more to the lack of strengthening of the surrounding muscles from inadequate conditioning than to increased ligamentous laxity. The only time women may be at in creased risk for ligamentous and musculoskeletal injuries is during the third trimester of pregnancy, when relaxing, a hormone that makes the pelvic area more flexible in preparation for delivery, is released, and all of the ligaments become more lax.

Stress Fracture

Stress fractures are pathologic fractures, partial or complete, in bone that has been weakened by long-term recurrent microtrauma. The major concerns about stress fractures in women relate to whether conditions such as amenorrhea, anorexia nervosa, low estrogen levels, and reduced calcium intake contribute to the pathologic fractures. Prolonged hypoestrogenism and low calcium intake are suspected to predispose women athletes to stress fractures.

This author studies 50 active women who had stress fractures, documented by x-ray and/or bone scan, identified retrospectively. There was no difference in the prevalence of haemorrhage in this group compared with a group of college athletes used as a control population. Most of the women were able to attribute their stress fractures to a change in training anatomy; equipment; environment; improper technique; or lack of conditioning. It is premature to relate stress fracture risk simply to haemorrhage. The duration of the haemorrhage, hypoestrogenemia, anorexia, low calcium intake, and the potential of earlier and more severe osteoporosis are all factors that merit further study.

Osteoporosis

Osteoporosis is characterized by decreased bone mass and increased susceptibility to fracture in the absence of other recognizable causes of bone loss. Clinical features include vertebral compression fractures, hip and wrist fractures.

Athletes who have poor nutrition, amenorrhea, and

anorexia need calcium supplementation and/or cyclic treatment with estrogen and progesterone. In the menstruating population of active/athletic women, weightbearing exercise has been shown to delay the onset and decrease the severity of osteoporosis. The issue of whether to treat postmenopausal women prophylactically and therapeutically is still controversial, but it is becoming clearer that treatment is indicated and should include estrogen-progesterone and calcium, or both, especially for those at risk.

Calcium

Bone accretion usually occurs until age 30-35, when peak bone mass is obtained. It has been noted in numerous articles that women's intake of calcium is much lower than the recommended 1000 mg for actively menstruating women and 1500 mg for non-menstruating and postmenopausal women. The best way to obtain calcium is from food, but if this is not possible because of weight restrictions, etc., calcium supplements should be added. Caffeine, alcohol, cigarette smoking, lactose intolerance, and fibre decrease the absorption, of calcium, as does as low estrogen level. Vitamin D and estrogens increase the absorption of calcium.

A practical guideline is that athletes who ingest less than 2,000 Kcal of calcium per day should have their diets supplemented with calcium and iron.

Amernorrheic and postmenopausal women should be trated with 0.625 mg estrogen per day on days 1-21 of the menstrual cycle, with the addition of progesterone, 10 mg/day on days 16-25. Amenorrheic young women can be cycled in this way every other month, so if their normal menstrual cycles resume both the doctor and patient will know it.

Vitamin D is obtained from sunlight and milk and, if necessary, may be supplemented with 400-800 units per day.

PSYCHOLOGY

Freud asked: "What does a woman want?" Bernstein and Warner respond: "Women want to be considered as separate, autonomous individuals with their own set of characteristics determined biologically and stemming from their early infantile relationships. They do not want these characteristics to be pejoratively labelled or considered to be merely a compensation for their damaged anatomy, not less good nor less desirable, or less important, merely different.

The Problem

"Assuming the young woman has the opportunity to participate in sports in the first place, the biggest problem she faces is the almost universal sterotype that say women are to be passive, dependent and emotional." Stark states, "The parents' social class can affect how a young girl perceives athletics; sports is rarely seen as a 'way out' even for lower socioeconomic class females, but being stereotypical female to attract a man is."

Corbin notes, "there is considerable evidence that may females lack self confidence in their abilities to perform sports and physical activities, especially in certain situations. This situational lack of confidence is most likely to occur in activities perceived to be sex-role inappropriate, in activities that are evaluative as well as competitive, and in situations in which performance feedback is lacking or unclear."